THE
WATER
WORKOUT
RECOVERY
PROGRAM

THE WATER WORKOUT RECOVERY PROGRAM

Safe and Painless Exercises for Treating Back Pain, Muscle Tears, Tendinitis, Sports Injuries, and More

ROBERT G. WATKINS, M.D.
Kerlan-Jobe Orthopaedic Clinic

BILL BUHLER
Head Trainer, Los Angeles Dodgers

and PATRICIA LOVEROCK

CB

CONTEMPORARY
BOOKS

CHICAGO · NEW YORK

Library of Congress Cataloging-in-Publication Data

Watkins, Robert G.
    The Water Workout Recovery Program : safe and painless
exercises for treating back pain, muscle tears, tendinitis, sports
injuries, and more / Robert G. Watkins, Bill Buhler, and Patricia
Loverock.
        256 pp.
    Bibliography: p. 236
    Includes index.
    ISBN 0-8092-4636-8 (pbk.) : $12.95
    1. Sports—Accidents and injuries—Exercise
therapy.   2. Aquatic exercises.   I. Buhler, Bill.   II. Loverock,
Patricia.   III. Title.
RD97.W38   1988
615.8′2—dc19   88-5078
                                                                         CIP

All photographs by Neilson Ayers except those on pages 6, 8,
and 19.
Illustrations by Lianne Auck.
Photographs on pages 6, 8, and 19 used with permission of the
Los Angeles Dodgers, Inc.

Published by Contemporary Books, Inc.
180 North Michigan Avenue, Chicago, Illinois 60601
Manufactured in the United States of America
Library of Congress Catalog Card Number: 88-5078
International Standard Book Number: 0-8092-4636-8

Published simultaneously in Canada by Beaverbooks, Ltd.
195 Allstate Parkway, Valleywood Business Park,
Markham, Ontario L3R 4T8 Canada

To our spouses, Katy, Barb, and Neil, for their love, encouragement, and good humor, and to all of the injured athletes who will find better health and peace of mind through water exercise.

Contents

Acknowledgments

The authors wish to thank the following individuals and organizations for their valuable assistance in the preparation of this book:

Lianne Auck, illustrator
Neil Ayers, photographer
Richard Bradford, Steve Bradford, Nora Clarke, Lee Eisler, Lynnsey Guerrero and Dave Stolzer, athlete models
The International Dance-Exercise Association
The Los Angeles Dodgers publicity department
Mike Marshall and Len Matuszek, players for the Los Angeles Dodgers
Kate Schmidt, hydrotherapist, International Sports Medicine Institute, Los Angeles, California, for sharing her expertise in water exercise
The Sherman family for the many times we used their pool
Kathy Williams, Dr. Watkins's helpful and patient secretary
And very special thanks to Nancy Smith Cox, registered physical therapist, Kerlan-Jobe Orthopaedic Clinic, without whose suggestions and dedication this book would not have been possible.

THE WATER WORKOUT RECOVERY PROGRAM

1
Introduction

During the past twenty-five years, America has become increasingly health and fitness conscious. It all started in the 1960s, largely due to the vitality and physical fitness of President John F. Kennedy. He believed that fifty-mile hikes and exercise in general must be part of the lives of all Americans, and he provided an example by playing sports himself. America was coming off a decade of having babies and enjoying the incredible post war relaxation, rejoicing, and prosperity. In the 1950s, Americans were recovering from the horrors of Hitler and Stalin and were sitting back to watch baseball, drink dry martinis, and smoke cigarettes. The fifties businessman was not a jogger. Maybe he mowed his lawn and coached Little League, but he seldom thought about the importance of his own physical fitness.

Then along came the vital, active, and energetic President Kennedy, who told us that America needed to get in shape. Later in the decade, fitness guru Dr. Kenneth

Cooper published his book *Aerobics,* and millions of Americans took up running. Now in the 1980s, exercising is a big part of our lives. According to a 1986 nationwide study by the National Sporting Goods Association, there are 49.7 million cyclists, 23.1 million runners, 21.9 million aerobic dancers, 21.2 million basketball players, 20.9 million softball players, 20.7 million volleyball players, and 12 million football players. And these participation figures are for just a few of the most popular sports and fitness activities in this country.

We have learned that exercise is good for our physical and mental health. It makes our heart and circulatory system stronger and gives us bigger muscles. It reduces our risk of heart disease, stroke, and cancer. It helps us lose weight and feel better about how we look. Our stress level is reduced and our sense of well being enhanced if we make exercise part of our weekly routine.

Is exercise all good? Nearly, but not quite. Sooner or later, exercise leads to injury, and injury is the dark side of exercise.

Sports- and fitness-related injuries have increased along with our activity levels. It is difficult to count how many sports-related injuries occur in this country every year, but the number is well into the millions. According to the National Athletic Trainers' Association estimates, one million high school athletes suffer injuries every year. In high school football alone, there are more than 600,000 "time loss" injuries—an injury that sidelines the player for at least one day—every year. Girls' interscholastic basketball, a sport that was seldom played back in the unfit days of the fifties and sixties, recorded approximately 126,000 injuries during the 1986–87 season. A study of hospital emergency rooms participating in a program called the National Electronic Injury Surveillance System estimated 1.4 million sports-related injuries were treated in these hospitals in 1985.

Why do these millions of injuries happen? A quick

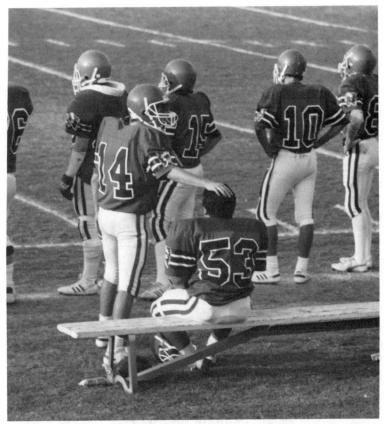

A teammate comforts an injured high school football player. More than 600,000 injuries occur every year in high school football.

survey of your friends who take part in sports will give you the answers. The following are some of the most common reasons you and your friends get hurt during exercise.

Overuse of Your Body

"Overuse injuries" are caused by doing too much too soon. These happen often to beginners who get inspired to take up a fitness activity or sport and don't give their body time to adapt to the higher level of physical activity. The body isn't used to the impact and stress of the sport, and it breaks. You strain a muscle, break a bone, or tear a ligament because you haven't taken the time to gradually build up the level of activity. Overuse injuries also happen to seasoned athletes who suddenly increase their workout load—for example, a runner increasing his mileage from thirty to fifty miles a week.

Improper Warm-Up

Your body needs to idle at low speed for a few minutes before you max it out. It takes only ten minutes of walking or jogging followed by a few simple stretches to prepare the body for more dynamic movement, but millions of exercisers don't have the patience to do a warm-up. They jump on the tennis court or into the softball game with little more than a quick toe touch. Then they go for the tough backhand or reach for the throw to first, and something gives. A muscle, tendon, or ligament rips, and the athlete is facing weeks of recovery that could have been avoided with a few minutes of easy warm-up.

Inadequate Footwear

The feet bear the brunt of sports participation. Proper athletic footwear will give the body the support it needs to run for home plate, to cut right to avoid a linebacker, or to land on hardwood after rebounding the basketball. Your shoes are the first line of defense against injury. Yet how many of us give them much thought? Those old reliable running shoes may look a little worn out, but they've still got lots of miles on them, right? Wrong. No matter what your sport, you should wear athletic shoes that support your feet properly. Proper athletic shoes are the most important piece of sports gear you own. Use them and abuse them; then lose them and get a new pair.

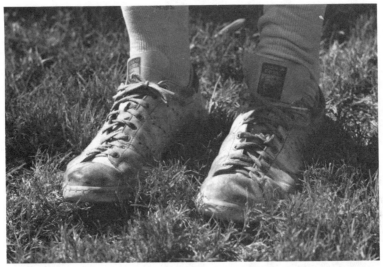

Exercising in old, worn-out athletic shoes such as these can lead to a sports injury.

Impact

Running into another player or a piece of equipment will obviously set you up for injury. There's nothing like meeting the boards in ice hockey or getting your body slammed by another player in football, baseball, or basketball to cause an injury. It happens all the time, and it often hurts.

These injuries happen, but if you treat them properly you'll be back in the game a lot faster. Water rehabilitation exercise is one of the best—but least understood—methods for getting better after a sports injury.

WHY SHOULD YOU FOLLOW A WATER RECOVERY PROGRAM?

If you've worked hard getting into shape and if you really love your sport, it can be discouraging to suddenly be rendered inactive because of an injury. You will want to do something to stay in shape, and you'll want to return to your dry-land exercise program as quickly as possible. Water exercise will let you accomplish both these goals. (We'll talk about fixing the mind along with the body in Chapter 3.)

Research has shown that you lose fitness twice as fast as you gain it. Let's say you've been exercising for two months and you've sprained your ankle. In four weeks you're going to be right back where you started *if you do no physical activity during your recovery time.* When your ankle is badly sprained—the most common sports injury—it may take that long before the swelling goes down and you can work out on land without pain. The pool gives you the key alternative. You can work out in water without hurting your ankle. You'll be able to maintain your level of fitness, keep your muscles strong and in tone, and actually speed your recovery from the sprain.

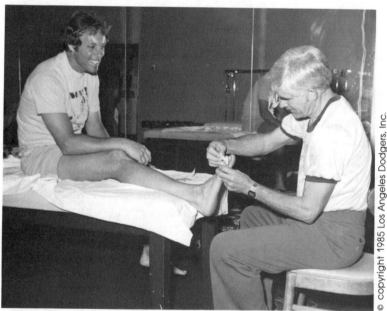

Former Los Angeles Dodger Jay Johnstone receives treatment from Bill Buhler. Bill's water recovery program is part of the daily exercise routine for injured players.

WHY DID WE WRITE THIS BOOK?

The use of water for relaxation and rehabilitation is not a new concept. The Romans had their baths, the ancient Greeks had the sea, and modern civilization has backyard and neighborhood swimming pools. Today, water is primarily thought of as a place to swim, frolic with the kids, or float on an air mattress and soak up the sun. But water exercise—workouts designed to tone your muscles and get your heart and lungs in shape—are being discovered as a fresh approach to fitness.

Water rehabilitation in a swimming pool is a fairly new idea. For about the past twenty years, physicians and physical therapists have been telling injured athletes to work out in the pool until their injuries have healed. But the "workout" has never really been defined. For some, working out means swimming laps. But many athletes find lap swimming boring and difficult. It's not an alternative for athletes who can't swim or those who are afraid of water. Telling an athlete to "use the pool" without assigning a specific workout usually means the pool exercise will be abandoned after two or three sessions. This book gives you a plan—goals and exercises—to help you stay with the recovery program until you are better and ready to return to your sport.

The exercises in this book are based on our experience working with athletes and rehabilitating our own sports injuries. We have talked to many athletes who have used the pool to recover from injury, and they have shared their ideas with us. These athletes represent the entire spectrum of sport, from Mike Marshall, the twenty-seven-year-old star slugger of the Los Angeles Dodgers, to Lynnsey Guerrero, a successful radio producer who likes to unwind from his job by running with his friends.

We discovered in our interviews and professional contact with these athletes that a water recovery pro-

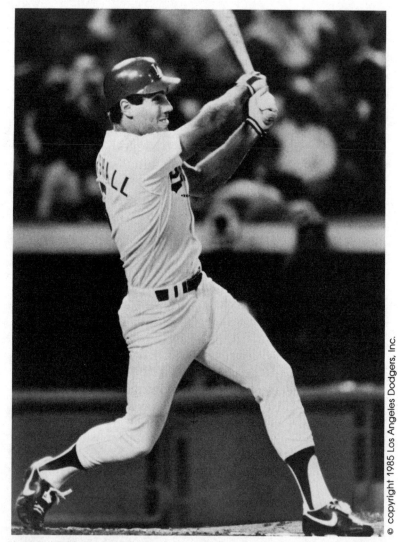

Los Angeles Dodger Mike Marshall was plagued by injuries during the 1987 season. Water exercise helped speed his recovery and enabled him to stay in good physical condition until he was ready to get back in the game.

gram works. We also discovered that in many cases the plan for these programs was hit and miss. It has usually been left up to the motivation and imagination of the injured person to come up with a workout. To take the guesswork out of water rehabilitation, we wanted to create a book that would establish an intelligent, safe, and effective workout program for the injured athlete during the weeks of recovery.

2
Why Work Out in Water?

The refreshing sensation you get when you jump into a pool, lake, or ocean is part of the joy of water exercise. It has a calming, relaxing effect on the body and at the same time is remarkably invigorating. But the pleasure of being in water is only part of what makes it the perfect place to exercise.

Water is virtually a risk-free exercise environment when it comes to joints, muscles, and bones. This is one of the reasons swimming has become the most popular sport in the country, with 72.6 million participants. When you are immersed in water, the body is about one-tenth as heavy as it is on dry land. If you weigh 160 pounds out of the water, you weigh only 16 underwater. Water is as close to zero gravity as you can get without traveling to outer space. Space shuttle astronauts learn how to operate equipment in space by training submerged in a 30-foot deep swimming pool.

The water exercises in this book don't take place totally underwater, but this doesn't mean you don't enjoy

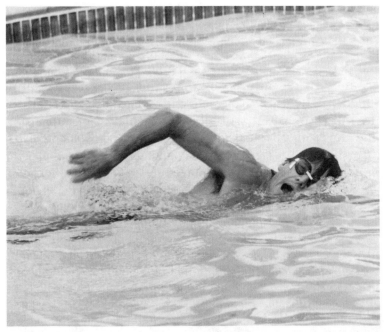

Swimming is one fitness activity that does not put stress on the joints, muscles, and bones. This is one reason why it is the most popular form of exercise in the country, with 72.6 million participants.

the benefits of water's support and buoyancy. Even when in neck- or chest-deep water, your weight is a fraction of what it is on land. Buoyancy allows you to exercise in water much sooner than on land. With the water supporting the muscles, joints, and bones around the injury, there is none of the impact stress that occurs when you exercise out of the water.

Exercising the injured part—strengthening and rehabilitating the area around the injury—can be done much more safely in the water, and this is what has made water rehabilitation so popular with physicians and physical therapists. A decade ago, doctors told the injured athlete to rest for a few weeks until the injury healed. Now we know that rest and inactivity may be the worst thing for an injury. The muscles atrophy and weaken, and the athlete loses physical condition and often becomes depressed and anxious. But for most injuries, normal exercise is not possible. Water exercise is the perfect alternative. A sensible water-exercise program will actually strengthen the injured part and speed the healing process by increasing circulation to the injured area. It will allow the athlete to maintain a high level of physical conditioning and a positive attitude during the recovery.

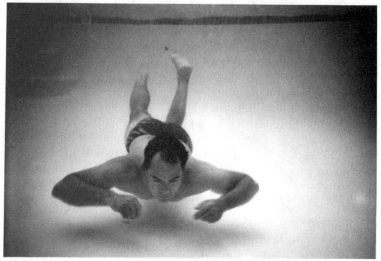

On dry land, this six-foot-six-inch athlete weighs 230 pounds. Submerged in the pool his body weight is about 23 pounds.

Water is a risk-free weight-training facility. As you move your body through the water, it resists your movement, causing your muscles to work harder. The natural resistance of water allows you to tone and strengthen muscles. The level of resistance is increased the faster you move your body against the water. This is why we suggest you move in a controlled, slow manner when first learning the exercises. As you become stronger, increase the speed of the moves, thereby increasing the resistance the water exerts on your muscles.

TALK TO YOUR PHYSICIAN

If the injury is checked by a physician, discuss a water rehabilitation program with the doctor before getting your feet wet. There may be movements that the physician will ask you to avoid. This doesn't mean you can't do the workout; just postpone some of the exercises until strength and mobility begin to return to the injured area.

If not under a physician's care, let pain be your guide. If the exercises cause you pain, don't do them. You will be able to start a water recovery program long before you are able to exercise without pain on land. If the exercise progression we have suggested is followed, you should experience no discomfort. But if an exercise *does* hurt, you are not ready for the exercise. If pain continues with movement or at rest for more than a week after the original injury, see a physician specializing in sports medicine. These specialists will understand the desire to stay active during recovery and will be supportive of your decision to do water exercise.

NONSWIMMERS CAN DO THIS PROGRAM

Many athletes are nonswimmers—some positively abhor exercising in water! But many of these people have successfully completed this program of water recovery. Bill Buhler has coached several Los Angeles Dodgers reluctant to get their feet wet. They simply didn't feel comfortable in the pool. Here are the steps Bill takes with these athletes. They will work for you as well.

1. Go to a pool that has a lifeguard. You will feel more secure knowing that there is a trained individual on hand to help you.

2. Don't work out alone. Find someone who can swim

with you. Make sure that person knows you are a nonswimmer or nervous in the water and that you may need their assistance.

3. Exercise in the shallow end. All of these exercises, with the exception of water running and cycling, are done in the shallow end. Even these deep end activities can be replaced with water walking or running in chest-deep water, providing the contact with the bottom does not aggravate your injury.

4. Wear a flotation device—even in the shallow end. Flotation will give you more confidence and control. A waterskiing belt, vest, or the specially designed Wet Vest® (see Chapter 13) are all excellent. The flotation device should allow you freedom of movement in the arms and legs. As you become more confident, you need not wear the flotation device unless in the deep end. But during the first few workouts, we suggest you wear it all the time.

5. Rather than doing exercises the first day, begin by walking back and forth in the shallow end. Your training partner should be at your side, lending confidence and encouragement. Once you feel relaxed and comfortable walking, try the exercises. Most athletes discover the sudden joy of painless movement and mobility overrides the fear of water after one or two sessions of walking.

Don't be embarrassed about your fear of the water. Lots of people feel the same way—even in the major leagues! They followed these steps and were able to overcome their fear. They went on to do a water recovery program that let them maintain fitness and return to their sport more quickly.

WHAT TO DO BEFORE YOU GET WET

The style of the pool, water temperature, and even your swimsuit can have a dramatic effect on the success of your water workout. Here are a few simple guidelines that will make your pool recovery program more convenient and enjoyable.

The Pool

You can use any size pool, from the Olympic to the backyard variety, as long as it has a shallow and a deep end. In a smaller pool, check out the slope of the bottom. It should be level where you are standing in chest-deep water. Sometimes small pools slope quickly toward the deep end, and it is difficult to maintain solid footing on the slanted bottom.

Once you have found a pool that is convenient and properly designed for your workout, make a note of the times it is available so you can plan a schedule. Then find another pool that meets your requirements, so you will have an alternate on days the first pool is closed.

Water Temperature

The most comfortable temperature for a pool workout is 82 to 84 degrees Fahrenheit. Water cooler than 78 degrees—like a mountain stream—will be bracing but too cold for you to enjoy the workout. Warmer than 90 degrees will be too warm. Try to find a pool that is within the range of 78 to 90 degrees Fahrenheit.

Your Swimsuit

Style is a big part of life, but so is comfort. Your swimsuit must be a practical design. For women, a one-piece racing style is the best. Stay away from high-cut legs or other styles that ride up the buttocks. Most bikinis are not suitable because they don't stay on during exercise. Men should wear a style that has strong elastic or a drawstring at the waist so the suit will stay put. Pick a fabric that is lightweight and fast drying. Polyester fabric is the most durable and chlorine resistant. Lycra Spandex suits are more lightweight and comfortable than polyester, but they tend to wear out more quickly in chlorine. Cotton, especially when it is blended with polyester, is comfortable and durable, but it does tend to stretch and lose shape. All fabric styles will last longer if you rinse your suit out in mild detergent after the workout. Read the manufacturer's label instructions for care and you will get a lot more wear out of the suit.

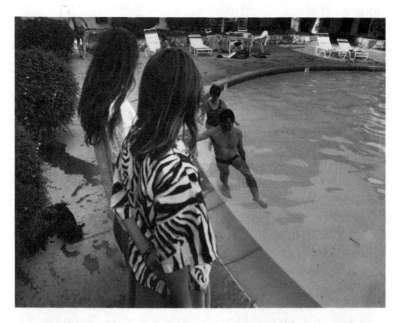

Curious onlookers, especially children, are bound to ask you about your water exercise program. Don't let their questions get in the way of your workout.

Attracting Attention

Experience teaches us that water exercise will draw attention to you in the pool. People will ask you what you are doing and why. Go ahead and tell them. A simple sentence, such as "I have a knee injury and I'm doing some pool exercises to get better," will satisfy their curiosity. Don't feel foolish if people stare or if kids try to follow along while you exercise. As soon as onlookers realize you are serious about what you are doing, they will respect your dedication and will actually offer you encouragement. Whatever you do, don't let long explanations and conversations get in the way of your workout.

Try not to place obstacles in your path to recovery. Even if the pool bottom isn't just right or the water is a bit cool or your swimsuit looks like something out of *Beach Blanket Bingo*, it's important to turn off the TV and go get yourself into the water. The choice is yours. Only you can decide whether you will do all you can to get better faster or settle for what may be a long and painful recovery.

3
Fixing the Mind and the Body

Dodger Len Matuszek, discussing his injury-plagued 1987 baseball season, had this to say: "I'm the kind of person that if I can't work out or train when I want to or need to, it causes me to become very depressed. When you can't perform, when you're an athlete who is hurt and can't go out there and play, do his job, and do what he is expected to do, that's a very rough time."

Late in April, Matuszek felt a nagging pain in his left foot. He thought it was nothing worth mentioning to the Dodger trainers. As Len puts it, "I'm not the kind of guy who comes and tells you when I have a hangnail." Like so many athletes, Matuszek is accustomed to playing with pain. A few days later, on April 30, during a game against the Pittsburgh Pirates, Len jumped to make a routine catch and his spikes tangled and snagged in the Astroturf carpet, but Len and his foot didn't stop. As he hobbled off the field, he knew that catch had pushed his foot over the edge. In fact, Len had ripped his plantar fascia, a sheath of connective tissue that lines the bot-

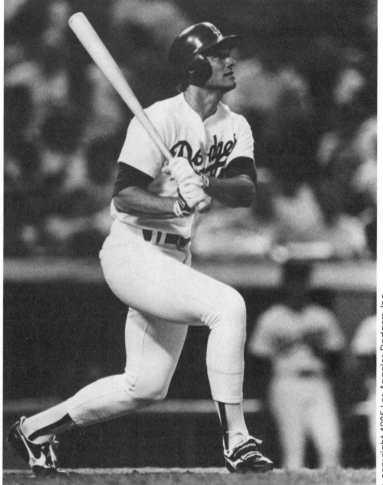

Dodger Len Matuszek at bat early in the 1987 season. A foot injury benched Len for most of the year. He maintained his physical and mental health with a daily water exercise program designed by Bill Buhler.

tom of the foot. Rather than facing opposing pitchers that season, Len faced surgery, hours of rehabilitation, and weeks of depression. Watching his team from the dugout was especially hard because the Dodgers were not having a great season.

"It's tough to just be sitting there, watching your teammates—your friends—going out there night after night, giving their best and coming up short. I hurt for them. I hurt for myself. I was going through every kind of emotion you can think of."

The psychological pain of an injury can be as hard to deal with as the physical hurt. For some athletes, especially those who suffer career-ending injuries, the psychological blow is much more difficult than the physical pain. And you don't have to be a major league player to experience the mental anguish of an injury. If you're hooked on a sport or fitness activity and suddenly can't do it, you're going to go through some mental adjustment.

How you deal with your emotional response to injury can make a big difference to recovery. Sports psychologists know that there is a fairly predictable pattern to what you are going to feel when injured. Understanding these emotional responses to injury will help you deal with them more easily. Some days, you are going to feel so down you'll cry. Other days, you'll throw your crutches across the room in anger. Know that these reactions are natural and normal. Millions of athletes have gone through the same upheaval.

THE EMOTIONAL SIDE OF INJURY

Sports psychologists say that an athlete's emotional reactions to an injury are similar to those that occur when a loved one dies. In her book *On Death and Dying*, psychologist Elisabeth Kübler-Ross described the emotional stages that occur with death. The reactions are, in order: disbelief, denial, isolation, anger, bargaining, depression, and acceptance.

Here's a sample of how this process might work when you have an athletic injury. You strain a ligament in your knee while sliding into home plate. At first you say to yourself: "This can't happen to me!"—*disbelief.* You tell your friends "Oh, it's nothing. It will be better in a day or two"—*denial.* Then, when the doctor tells you it is serious and you will have to sit out competition and training, you feel alone and lonely—*isolation.* You become irritated and angry with yourself and those around you, thinking "How could this happen to me?"—*anger.* After a few days of rehabilitation, you tell the doctor you will take it easy in the game if he'll just give you the okay to play—*bargaining.* He orders you to stick to your rehab program, and you go home to sit in front of the television and sink into a deep funk—*depression.* Finally, after a few days of this, you resign yourself to several weeks of physical therapy, realizing that's the only way you'll get back in the game—*acceptance.*

"MAYBE I'LL JUST TEST IT"

Of all these stages, the denial phase may be the most dangerous. World renowned sports psychologist Dr. Bruce Ogilvie explained in an interview for this book that during the denial phase you may do things that will make your injury worse. The athlete may take pain medication (we talk about the danger of that strategy later) or may just exercise with the pain, hoping the problem isn't that serious. This attitude can lead to much more serious injuries, says Ogilvie, and even permanent damage to the body. Len Matuszek admits now that he may have saved himself from the more serious injury if he had just mentioned the nagging pain in his foot to the Dodger trainers before he started the game against the Pirates.

Denial can manifest itself in seemingly innocent ways. Imagine, for example, that you've sprained your ankle. It's pretty bad, but you've been off it for a week. You go out to the game and tell yourself, "Maybe I'll just throw the ball around a little, just to test the ankle." Reaching for the ball, your ankle twists and your brain screams with pain. You've just set recovery back another week, perhaps longer. The phrase "I just thought I'd test it to see if it was OK" may be the most common lament among injured—and then reinjured—athletes. Denying the injury won't make it go away.

COPING STRATEGIES

There are a lot of things that will help you cope with the mental challenge of injury rehabilitation. The water exercises in this book are an excellent starting point. This program is good for your mental health because it lets you exercise, and inactivity is one of the most depressing aspects to any injury. Len Matuszek says he was really hitting bottom before Bill Buhler approached him about trying a water recovery program that would help his foot and maintain his fitness during the weeks of recovery. At first he was hesistant. "I'm not a strong swimmer," explained Len. But Bill gave him a flotation device and coached him throughout his daily workouts.

"When I was able to exercise and work out in the pool, my mental state improved so much I actually felt good," said Matuszek.

According to sports psychologists Dr. Robert J. Rotella and Dr. Steven R. Heyman, there are other valuable coping strategies that will help you reduce the psychological stress an athletic injury may create. Use these techniques to avoid postinjury psych-outs.

Knowledge

Seek out honest and accurate information about the injury. Find out what has been hurt and why. If you are going to have surgery, talk to the surgeon about the procedure and why it is necessary. You will be less anxious and less likely to deny the severity of the injury if you understand what is really happening to your muscles, tendons, ligaments, and joints.

Each exercise chapter in this book starts with an explanation of the physiology of the body part you will be exercising. Then there is a description of the major injuries and reasons why water exercise will speed your recovery. Read the pages that apply to your injury. The more you know about the body and the part you have hurt, the more motivated you will be to continue with the recovery program. If you don't know why you do a program of rehabilitation—including this one—it is easy to doubt its value and to abandon it. Knowledge is your safeguard against denial, and it will give you a positive attitude about your recovery program.

Imagery

You will need to have a detailed understanding of your injury for this to be effective. Imagine the positive effect your water recovery exercises are having on your injury. Visualize the healing process. Think about how the muscles are becoming stronger and how the stress on your bones and muscles is reduced in the water.

You're Only Human

Tell yourself that you are not weak willed or physically inadequate because you are injured. Sports injuries happen to millions every year. It's normal and reasonable to feel frustrated, angry, and disappointed that you cannot take part in sports.

Self-Talk

A recovery program is not as exciting as your regular workouts, so it is easy to gripe. Try to turn these negative thoughts into positive thoughts. Tell yourself, "This

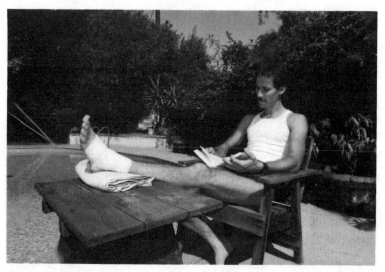

If you understand your injury, you'll be more likely to stick with your rehabilitation program. Spend some of your recovery time reading and learning about your injured body part.

is like watching paint dry, but I'll stick with it. At least I get to exercise, and it's helping me get back to competing again." Your inner dialogue is very important to the success of your recovery.

STICKING WITH IT

Water exercise probably isn't nearly as much fun as the sport that injured you. There are going to be times when you will feel like staying home or (worse) doing some activity that will create a risk of reinjury. Here are some simple steps that will keep you in the pool and on the road to recovery.

1. Find a training partner. It is a lot more fun to train with someone, so find one or two reliable people to be your training partner. A training partner will give you a soul mate against curious onlookers. A buddy will give you encouragement, and you'll be more

likely to get to the pool if your partner is counting on you. *Nonswimmers must exercise with a buddy who can swim, or exercise at a pool with a lifeguard.*

Your training partner doesn't have to be an adult. Many athletes we interviewed told us that they took their own children with them to the pool—children who already knew how to swim. The athletes did the workout, and the children either joined them or played on their own in the water. The kids enjoy it and are real motivators. Anyone with children knows that once you've promised to take a child to the pool, it's not easy to back out of the deal.

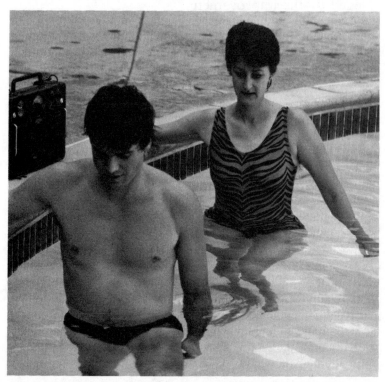

A reliable, encouraging training partner will help motivate you to do your pool exercises, especially on days you're feeling depressed about your injury.

2. Set reasonable goals. Recovery from an injury takes time. Sometimes improvement is measured by a fraction-of-an-inch increase in a joint's range of movement, or by the fact you can walk across the pool twice rather than just once. Your recovery may take weeks. Don't look for drastic improvement from day to day. Talk to your physician about your recovery and the kind of progress you can expect. Keep a training diary, noting the sets and reps you do each day and how the injury feels. Did you try an exercise that you could not do because of pain? Write it down and try it again in a week. After two or three weeks you will look back on your progress and be encouraged by the improvement.

3. Establish a routine. One of the keys for sticking with any program is making it a regular part of your schedule. Set a time for your workout and stick with it.

A FEW WORDS ON PAIN

You should not do any exercise that causes pain due to the injury. Sometimes that pain is felt at the injury site, but you may experience referred pain, which is created by the injury but felt in a different part of the body. Get to know what is "your pain"—the pain you felt when the injury occurred—and don't ignore your pain when you are exercising. If it hurts, don't do the movement.

Of course, as you probably know, any new form of exercise, even this water recovery program, will cause muscle stiffness and soreness. When you use muscles that may have been weakened due to inactivity—especially if you've had a prolonged layoff because of the injury—there is going to be some stiffness. Even if you're perfectly fit, new sports and exercises work muscles in new ways, and it takes time for the body to tone up to these new actions. The muscles may hurt the day after exercise because you have pushed them a little harder than normal. Stiffness and soreness of this variety is not harmful. It simply means you are making your muscles stronger, which is the point of this program.

NARCOTIC PAIN KILLERS

The use of narcotic medications, such as codeine, oxycodone, and morphine, is not recommended as a way to decrease your pain and enhance your rehabilitation program. They don't work well for long-term chronic pain caused by a serious sports injury. This is because the body has pain-eliminating chemicals that it normally produces itself. Narcotics block the production of these chemicals. When the narcotics are depleted in the system, the nerves are left raw with no natural defense against pain. You have a wide-open circuit for pain and need more narcotics to ease the pain, and the cycle continues. You can easily wind up with an intrusive, unhealthy, expensive, and even illegal drug addiction that will be difficult to overcome and not do very much for your sports injury. Patients who have taken narcotics for extended periods to ease their pain say routinely that they don't enjoy the medication. It's just that they can't stand the pain without the drugs.

Narcotics will also increase the risk of your doing too much too soon and making the injury worse. When the pain centers are completely blocked, you can move in a way that will damage your body. The alternative is to stay off an injury that hurts so much you need narcotics. If you have chronic pain, see a physician. If a movement hurts your injury, don't take a pill so you can do the movement! Cut back on your activity until you can do it in a pain-free way.

The water exercises described in this book will stimulate the production of your natural painkilling chemicals. If you are stiff or sore before your workout, you may find you feel much better after a few minutes in the pool.

4
Planning Your Water Recovery Workout

The next few pages contain the most important information in this book. Read it once, then read it again. The most challenging aspect to your water recovery program is knowing how to plan your workout. The following guidelines will permit you to make sensible decisions about the intensity and progression of your water recovery program.

IF IT HURTS, DON'T DO IT!

You may wonder whether you should do a certain exercise or add more exercises to your program. Only you can tell if an exercise is right for you, and the important rule to follow here is: *don't do it if it causes pain.* You can't work through pain and make yourself better. This kind of attitude can only aggravate your injury. Pain is your body's way of telling you to stop. Listen to your body.

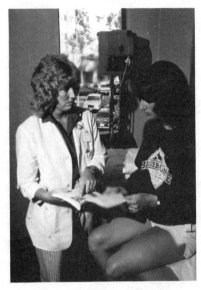

If you are under the care of a physician or physical therapist, discuss the water exercises in this book with that person before you begin your workouts.

GETTING STARTED

If you are under the care of a physician, trainer, or physical therapist, we strongly suggest you show these exercises to that person before you start your workout. Talk over whether or not you are ready to start this exercise program. If you are free of the symptoms of your injury when you are not bearing weight, chances are you can handle these exercises. If you have had surgery, you can usually begin your water exercise program as soon as the cast and/or stitches are removed. But you should check with your physician first.

If you are caring for your injury yourself—not an uncommon situation with many sports injuries—you will have to let pain be your guide. You will be able to start these exercises before you can tolerate weight-bearing activity such as walking or running. But if your injury is painful when you do these exercises, you shouldn't start the program. You may want to give yourself three or four days' rest, staying off the injury, before you begin. By then you should have no pain when doing the beginning-level water exercises. If the exercises still cause pain after one week, you should see a physician, preferably someone who specializes in treating sports injuries.

EXERCISE ORDER

The exercises are shown in ascending order of difficulty. The first one is less challenging to your injured part than the second and so on. During your first week, start with the water cycling or water jogging warm-up shown at the end of this chapter, followed by three exercises. *Don't overdo it.* Add one or two exercises a week until you are doing each exercise that is listed in the section that pertains to your injury. Remember, never do an exercise if it causes pain.

DURATION OF YOUR WATER RECOVERY PROGRAM

This program is designed to be done for just six to eight weeks. By that time you will be well and wanting to get back to your sport. These exercises are an important middle step between the day your injury put you on the sidelines and the day you do your first postrecovery workout in your sport. This program is part of the gradual rebuilding you must do to be sure you don't get injured again.

Now that we've said that, we should also say that many injured athletes continue doing water exercise once they have returned to their sport. In particular, the aerobic conditioning workouts shown in chapter 11 offer a nonimpact form of exercise that is a welcome alternative to running. Not that you need to give up your running workouts altogether. The athletes who do water running find that just doing a small percentage of their workouts in the pool reduces their injury rate.

THE WORKOUT INTENSITY

The one word you should think of when you are doing this program is "cadence." The speed with which you move your limbs through the water determines the amount of resistance you are working against. If you move quickly, your muscles must work harder. If you move slowly, the muscles can relax a little. Altering this cadence will greatly change the difficulty of your workout.

Obviously, you should start with slow movements. As the weeks progress, you can gradually increase the speed, or cadence, of your movements and thereby increase the level of strength you are building up in the injured area. If you move too quickly too soon, you risk stressing the injury beyond a healthy point. We recommend the first few repetitions of the exercise be done very slowly; you will learn your level of tolerance as well as the position your body should be in for the exercise.

CONCENTRATE!

Notice that in the workout schedule we recommend you do a maximum of four sets of ten repetitions for each exercise. One repetition is one completion of a movement. A set is used to describe the number of times you do the repetition without stopping. For example, two sets of ten repetitions of sit-ups means you have done ten sit-ups without stopping, rested for a few seconds, and then done ten more.

Some exercises require that you work the right side of the body separately from the left. In these cases, complete ten repetitions on one side and then ten on the other. This equals one set. (The maximum number of repetitions you will do is forty per side.)

Each exercise description tells you what comprises one repetition for that exercise. If you do ten repetitions, you have completed one set.

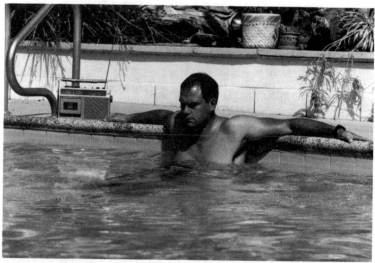

As you do each repetition, concentrate on maintaining correct body position and exercise techniques. Move in a slow, controlled manner.

There is a good reason we ask you to do a maximum of only four sets of ten repetitions of each exercise. We want you to concentrate on your body position and the movement of your body in the water. Too many repetitions of one exercise without a break will cause you to lose concentration. Your exercise technique will suffer, and that's not good for the injury. Think about each repetition as you go through the movement and ask yourself these questions:

Is your body in the correct position?
Are you compensating for your injury by using a different part of your body?
Does it hurt while you're doing the exercise?
Does the injury feel better as you do the exercise?

Once you can handle four sets of ten reps, increase the difficulty of the exercise by increasing the speed with which you do the movement. Your goal, however, should always be quality, not quantity. Concentrate on your form and technique no matter how fast you think you can do the movement.

EXERCISE BOTH SIDES OF YOUR BODY

It is important that you do the exercise on both sides of your body, not just the side that is injured. If you have a hamstring pull in the right leg, do the movements with both your right and your left leg. This will allow you to maintain muscle balance, which will help prevent reinjury.

LEARN ABOUT YOUR INJURY

We have prefaced each of the exercise sections with a description of the part of the body you will be using during the movements and the most common injuries to that body part. We believe that the more you know about your body and the injury, the easier it will be to understand why you are doing a certain exercise. This kind of knowledge will help keep you motivated to stay with your rehabilitation program. Sports psychologists have determined that the more an athlete knows about the injury, healing process, and reasons for the rehabilitation program, the greater the chance that the athlete will stick with it. Read the few pages about your body so you can understand your injury, the healing process, and how this water recovery program will help you.

WRAP YOUR WORKOUT

The poolside is not the best place for this book, or any other for that matter. Before long it will be soggy, wrinkled, and unreadable. You will have to use plastic to protect your workout. Since we have included a sum-

mary of the exercises at the end of each chapter, pho-
tocopy those pages and the workout schedule also
listed. Slip the copy into a plastic bag. The type that zips
closed at the top works very well. Stationery stores sell
clear plastic pockets designed to protect a sheet of pa-
per, and these are also excellent at pool side.

WATER WARM-UP

Before you begin your water exercise program, do one of these warmups.

Water Cycling

This warm-up is for injuries to the foot, ankle, knee, thigh, hip, buttocks, and back. It may also be used for shoulder, wrist, and elbow injuries.

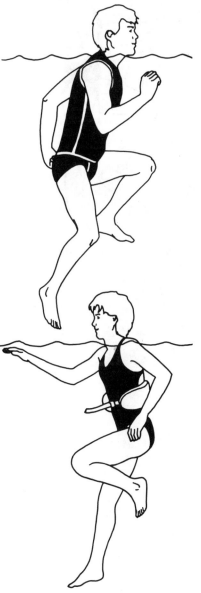

While wearing a flotation device, such as a waterskiing belt, vest, or the Wet Vest, go into the deep end, gently move your legs in a cycling motion. It is easier to keep your head above water if you keep your hands in the cupped position. Move your arms back and forth, as if you are running slowly. You may find yourself bending at the waist, so concentrate on keeping your body upright in the water. Continue for five minutes.

Note: You can maintain your aerobic conditioning during your recovery by doing a program of water running. Rather than running your mileage or interval training on land, you can duplicate your program in the pool. Please turn to chapter 11 for information on water workouts for aerobic conditioning.

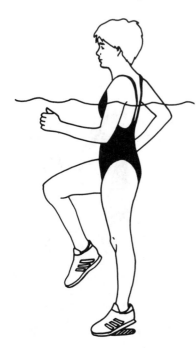

Water Jogging

This warm-up may be used for injuries to the shoulder, wrist, and elbow if you choose not to do water cycling. (This weight-bearing warm-up will not jeopardize these parts of the body.)

Stand in chest-deep water. Run slowly from one side of the pool to the other. Continue for five minutes.

Note: You may find it more comfortable to wear a pair of athletic shoes during this warm-up.

Turn now to the section dealing with your injury and familiarize yourself with the exercises you will be doing.

WORKOUT SCHEDULE

This program is designed to last six to eight weeks, the length of time it usually takes to recover from an injury.

Weeks 1 and 2

Frequency: Do the exercises three days a week with at least one rest day between training sessions.

Intensity: Do water warm-up and the first three exercises in the section dealing with your injury.

Duration: Do two sets of 10 repetitions for each exercise.

Weeks 3 and 4

Frequency: Do the exercises five days a week with two rest days. Don't take two rest days in a row.

Intensity: Do water warm-up. In addition to the three exercises you did in weeks 1 and 2, add two exercises each week to the program.

Duration: Do three sets of 10 repetitions for each exercise.

Weeks 5 to 8

Frequency: Do the exercises six days a week. Take one rest day.

Intensity: Do water warm-up. In addition to the exercises you did in week 4, add one or two exercises each week until you are doing all the movements shown in the section dealing with your injury.

Duration: Do four sets of 10 repetitions for each exercise.

5
Feet, Ankles, and Lower Legs

Just as the world's finest-handling performance car wouldn't be much good with four old, worn-out tires, so the best athlete is severely limited when a foot is injured. Everyday activities place considerable stress on the foot, but if you are an athlete, the stresses and strains on your feet are multiplied many times over. When you run at a moderate pace, your feet strike the ground with an impact that is up to five times your body weight. If you cut quickly on Astroturf or explode off the ground to clear a high-jump bar or rebound a basketball, the stress on your feet is incredible. Is it any wonder that foot injuries are so common in athletics?

There are twenty-six bones in each foot and a myriad of ligaments that link these bones to each other. The muscles of the lower leg are joined to the ankle and bones of the feet by tendons, the tough connective tissue that joins muscle to bone. You might think that with all of these parts, a lot can go wrong with the system, but it is the complex way that these parts work together that keeps the foot doing its job. The bones, ligaments, and tendons slide and turn as you walk, jump, run, and impact upon the ground; it's a sophisticated suspension and shock-absorption system. But when this system is abused by overuse (a common problem with long-distance runners), inadequate athletic footwear, or trauma, it breaks down.

The ankle joint is a hinge joint allowing you to flex the foot (raise it upward) and extend it (point it downward). It is created by the meeting of the tibia and fibula, the bones in your shin, with the talus, a large bone at the top of your foot. These three bones fit together very well, much like a flexible dovetail joint, and they are strapped in place by ligaments. Just below the ankle, the talus forms a joint with the calcaneus, or heel bone. This joint allows you to roll your foot inward and outward and, like the ankle, is supported by ligaments. These two joints work together with the bones of the feet to move the foot through its full range of motion.

This flexible dovetail joint of the ankle and its rotating neighbor joint just below would have few problems if you never asked them to go beyond their normal range of motion. Unfortunately, sports puts these joints in a precarious position, and all too often the foot is forcefully turned to one side or the other, such as when you step in a hole or twist your foot when you land. The ligaments around the bones become stretched or torn, and you've got a sprained ankle. There are no supporting muscles around the ankle and heel, so the ligaments that join the bones to each other bear the brunt of this common and painful injury.

The shinbones, the tibia and fibula, are the support structure for the lower leg. They too carry you through miles of running, working as a team with the foot to propel you through your athletic activities. The muscles on the front of the lower leg, the extensor digitorum longus, extensor hallucis longus, tibialis anterior, and peroneus tertius, pass over the top of the ankle and are

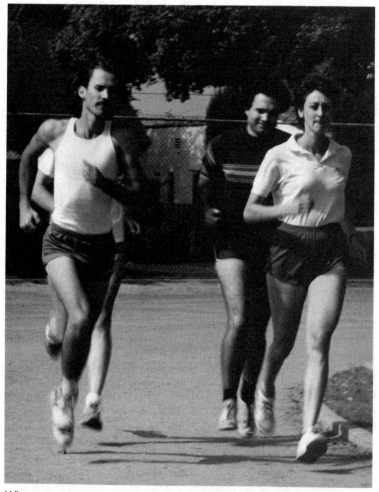

When you run, your foot strikes the ground with a force three to five times your body weight. This is one of the reasons foot, ankle, and lower-leg injuries are so common in this sport.

linked by tendons to the foot. Their major job is to keep the foot elevated as you walk, an important task indeed—you wouldn't get far if your foot flopped and dragged on the ground every time you tried to take a step. Some of these muscles are also responsible for allowing your ankle to roll outward, or supinate. The gastrocnemius, which gives the calf its rounded shape, is the most obvious of the six muscles that form the back of the lower leg. The calf muscles extend your ankle joint so you can point your toe, which is why they are well developed in ballerinas and gymnasts. The muscles on the outside of the lower leg, the peroneus longus and brevis, allow your ankle to pronate, or roll inward. These muscles on the back and sides of the lower leg attach to the foot by sneaking around and under the prominent ankle bones. This is why, if you have weakness or injury in the lower leg muscles, you may feel pain in the tendons of your foot.

WATER EXERCISE FOR FOOT, ANKLE, AND LOWER LEG INJURIES

This water rehabilitation program is a perfect way to maintain your strength and speed your recovery from an injury in these areas. The first thing any sports medicine specialist will tell you after an injury to the foot, ankle, or lower leg is to get off your feet. As long as you are forcing your injury to bear weight, it is not going to get better. Getting off your feet may mean using crutches or even a wheelchair for a while, but these encumbrances don't mean you can't use the pool. In the water, not only will you be off your feet, but you will be able to maintain your strength and fitness without further stressing your injury.

Athletes often make the mistake of thinking that an ankle or foot injury isn't as serious as those in other parts of the body. Not true! These injuries usually cause you to limp, favoring one leg over the other. Changing your gait to lessen pain can lead to pain and injury in the knee, thigh, hip, and even your back. This is one of the reasons a physician will tell you to get off your feet until the injury has healed. In the water, especially when you do noncontact movements such as the ones shown here, you will not have to compensate for your injury. You will use both sides of your body equally, thereby eliminating the risk of further injuries.

COMMON FOOT, ANKLE, AND LOWER LEG INJURIES

The exercises in this program are designed to rehabilitate the following foot, ankle, and lower leg injuries and to strengthen the involved muscles.

Plantar Fasciitis (Heel Spur)

The plantar fascia is part of your foot's suspension system. It is a fibrous connective tissue that runs along the bottom of the foot and inserts into the heel bone. With overuse, the fascia can become inflamed at the point where it attaches to the heel bone. As the injury progresses, the pain can spread over the bottom of the foot. Runners who are putting in too much mileage without enough recovery time or who suddenly increase their mileage are likely candidates for plantar fasciitis.

Bone Bruise

This injury usually starts with inadequate footwear. The lining around the small bones of the foot becomes inflamed after you step on a stone or other small, hard object. The bruise can last for weeks if you don't take a break from your sport and take the pressure off the foot bones.

Plantar Neuroma (Morton's Neuroma)

A neuroma is a tumor that forms around nerve fibers. In this case, the tumor forms between your toes because of constant compression on the nerve. The compression may be caused by wearing shoes that are tight fitting, such as the racing spikes worn by sprinters. If your foot rolls inward (pronates) excessively, compression can also occur when you run. If conservative measures—such as rest and wearing orthotics, specially designed shoe inserts—don't take away the pain, you may need surgery to remove the tumor.

Stress Fractures of the Foot Bones

Constant pounding of the feet, usually from running, can cause tiny fractures in the bones of the feet. The most common site for this injury is the large toe bones, or metatarsals. Once you have the fracture, you will need to stop doing your sport, especially workouts involving running and jumping, until the fracture heals. Your physician may put you on crutches or in a cast.

Sesamoiditis and Sesamoid Stress Fracture

Sesamoid bones are those that sit inside tendons rather than connecting to other bones via ligaments. There are sesamoid bones in the tendon underneath your big toe, and they are there to distribute the weight of your body as you propel yourself forward or jump. The tendon around the bone can become inflamed with overuse, a condition known as sesamoiditis. Continued stress may cause the bone to fracture. Gymnasts and dancers are prone to these injuries because these athletes repeatedly land on the balls of their feet, which puts continued stress on the sesamoids.

Lateral and Medial Ankle Sprains

This is the most common injury in sports. About 80 percent of all ankle sprains occur on the outer, or lateral, side of the ankle because the structure of the joint allows the foot to roll outward more easily than inward. A poorly placed step can cause you to turn your ankle as you land; your foot rolls outward far beyond the range of motion of the ankle joints, and ligaments that attach to the bones on the outside of the ankle are stretched or torn.

Medial sprains, ones in which the ligaments on the inner side of the joint are stretched or torn, are much more rare than lateral sprains, but they can be more serious. It takes a great deal of force to turn the ankle inward. For example, a football or baseball player running at top speed suddenly plants his foot and changes direction but his cleats stick in the turf. The leg continues in the direction of the player's move, but the foot remains firmly planted, forcing the ankle to roll inward. Not only are the ligaments strained or torn, but the force may actually fracture the end of the fibula.

A sprained ankle must be fully healed before you return to athletics or you risk permanent instability of the joint. Strengthening the lower leg muscles—as the exercises in this chapter do—will help prevent future sprains.

Achilles Tendinitis

The Achilles tendon is the largest, strongest tendon in the body. It connects the gastrocnemius muscle in the calf to your heel bone. If your large calf muscle is tight, a common problem with long-distance runners and jumpers, the stress of activity is transferred to the tendon. Unlike muscles, tendons can't stretch very far, and when they are forced beyond their capacity, microscopic tears occur. The tendon becomes inflamed and sore, especially during the first few minutes of your workout. Tears may also develop in the sheath of connective tissue that surrounds the tendon, again causing pain and inflammation.

It is important to nip this injury in the beginning

stages. If you ignore it and continue to tear either the tendon or the sheath, scar tissue begins to form and eventually you may need surgery to repair the damage. Since this injury is caused by overuse, your symptoms should disappear with sufficient rest. The pain will return, however, if you don't build your workouts gradually. Water exercises will allow you to maintain your fitness and build strength while the tendon heals.

Shin Splints

This injury plagues many beginning exercisers. The muscles on the front of the lower leg become sore and stiff, especially near the shinbone. The pain is caused by microscopic tears in the muscle fibers or the connective tissue that joins these muscles to the bone. The tearing occurs because you try to do too much exercise too soon, which is why the enthusiastic beginner gets shin splints. Runners who put in too many miles and aerobic dancers who take too many classes are likely candidates for shin splints, especially if these athletes have been inactive for a number of years. You will need to cut back on your workouts and strengthen the muscles of the lower leg. These water exercises will help you stay on the road to fitness, without aggravating your injury.

Rupture of the Achilles Tendon

Persistent Achilles tendinitis can so weaken the tendon that it actually ruptures. Usually it happens after you have done a sudden, forceful contraction of the calf muscles. Older athletes who have had sore Achilles tendons for years may suffer this injury. You stretch for a forehand in tennis or leap to make a shot in basketball and the tendon gives. Oddly enough, this rupture doesn't cause much pain but you will hear a "pop" when it happens. You may not know you have been injured—that is, until you try to stand on your toes and realize you can't because the tendon is no longer attached to the calf muscles.

Surgery is usually necessary to reattach the tendon. Check with your surgeon before you start water exercise because postsurgery management of this injury is usually quite cautious. You'll probably have to take it easy for a while.

Stress Fractures of the Lower Leg

Overuse, usually from running or jumping without a gradual buildup in a workout schedule, may cause tiny fractures to occur on the bones in the lower leg. The tibia is the most common location, but sometimes these fractures occur on the fibula, especially if you are a beginning runner. When you exercise, the bones actually increase in density to handle the stress. This building process takes time, and if you stress the bones too much before they have adapted to the level of activity, stress fractures form.

You'll first notice the injury as a tiny sore spot on the surface of the bone. If you continue doing a high level of activity, the fracture will increase in size and eventually you will have to stop your sport. Obviously, the best thing to do is catch a stress fracture early and cut back on your workouts. These water exercises will help you maintain your lower leg strength without putting further stress on the bone. A few days of water exercise may give the bone enough time to heal and become stronger—if you catch the stress fracture when it is still small. Otherwise, you may be looking at several weeks of rest and rehabilitation.

Gastrocnemius Tear (Tennis Leg)

This injury is more common among middle-aged athletes, especially if the calf muscles are tight or weakened by a previous injury. It occurs when you suddenly straighten your leg while the foot is firmly planted on the ground, such as when you reach for a forehand on the tennis court. The large calf muscle tears and you may require surgery to repair the damaged tissue. Depending on the degree of the tear, your recovery may take several weeks. You can begin these water rehabilitation exercises when your cast is removed or when your physician says you are ready for mild exercise. If you begin too soon, you risk reinjury.

THE EXERCISES

Never do exercises that cause pain in the joint, especially at the site of your injury. Follow the workout guidelines presented in chapter 4.

Warm-Up
Water Cycling, as described on page 35.

Noncontact Movements

Exercises 1 through 5 can be done sitting on the edge of the pool with legs dangling in the water. You may also sit on the stairs leading into the pool or on a plastic chair or milk crate in the shallow end. If your injury hurts when you stand, walk, or run, begin your water rehabilitation program with these noncontact movements.

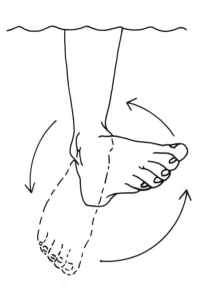

I. Foot Circles
Body parts strengthened: foot (extensor digitorum brevis, intrinsic plantar flexors); front and sides of lower leg (tibialis anterior, extensor digitorum longus, extensor hallucis longus, peroneus longus and brevis); calf (tibialis posterior, flexor digitorum longus, flexor hallucis longus, gastrocnemius, soleus).

Sit on the pool edge, dangling your legs in the water. Slowly turn your left foot in a clockwise circle, moving it with the ankle joint only. One turn equals one repetition. Do five turns clockwise, then five turns counterclockwise. Repeat with the right foot. This equals one set.

2. Ankle Flexions and Extensions

Body parts strengthened: foot (extensor digitorum brevis, intrinsic plantar flexors); front and sides of lower leg (tibialis anterior, extensor digitorum longus, extensor hallucis longus, peroneus longus and brevis); calf (tibialis posterior, flexor digitorum longus, flexor hallucis longus, gastrocnemius, soleus).

Sit on the pool edge with your legs in the water. Point the toes of your right foot toward the bottom, then toward the surface. This is one repetition. Ten with the right foot followed by ten with the left equals one set.

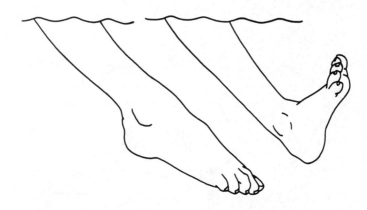

3. Alphabet

Body parts strengthened: foot (extensor digitorum brevis, intrinsic plantar flexors); front and sides of lower leg (tibialis anterior, extensor digitorum longus, extensor hallucis longus, peroneus longus and brevis); calf (tibialis posterior, flexor digitorum longus, flexor hallucis longus, gastrocnemius, soleus).

Sit on the edge of the pool with your legs dangling in the water. Using the big toe of your right foot as a "pen" write the first ten letters of the alphabet—A through J—in the water. Keep your lower leg still. Use only your ankle joint, not your knee or hip joints, while writing with your foot. One letter equals one repetition. Repeat with the other foot. Ten letters with the right foot followed by ten with the left equals one set.

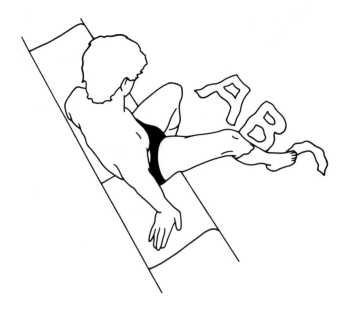

4. Soccer Kicks

Body parts strengthened: front of lower leg (tibialis anterior, extensor digitorum longus, extensor hallucis longus); front of thigh (quadriceps); back of thigh (hamstrings).

Sit on the edge of the pool with your legs dangling in the water. Flex both feet toward your body and turn them slightly inward. Holding the foot in this position, slowly kick one leg out and then the other. As you kick, keep your feet and lower legs in the water. Raise each foot to a point at which it is just below the surface. One kick of each leg equals one repetition.

Precaution: Keep the foot flexed when doing this movement, especially if you have an ankle sprain. If the foot flops around in the water as you do the kicks, you may aggravate the sprained ligaments. This flexed position will increase the resistance of the water, which in turn will increase the strengthening of the muscles on the front of the calf.

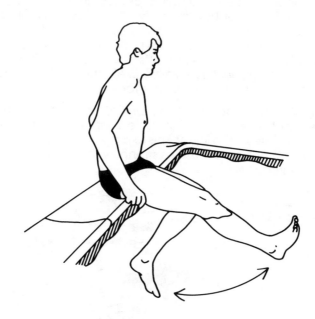

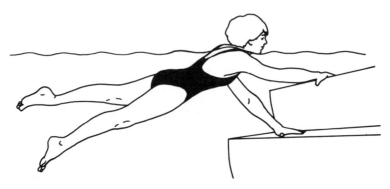

5. Straight-Leg Kicks

Body parts strengthened: hip (iliopsoas, sartorius, tensor fascia lata); inner thigh (adductor longus, brevis, and magnus; gracilis; pectineus); back of thigh (hamstrings); buttocks (gluteus maximus).

If the pool you are using has steps, float in the prone position and place your hands on the steps. If your pool does not have steps, float in the prone position, grip the side of the pool with one hand, and brace yourself with the other hand by turning it downward, as shown. *Kick your legs from the hip, keeping your knees straight.* Alternate left and right. One kick of each leg equals one repetition.

Note: An injury to the foot, ankle, or lower leg may weaken all the leg and hip muscles, especially if the pain makes you "favor" the injury. This exercise lets you keep your leg, hip, and buttocks muscles strong, without putting stress on the injured area.

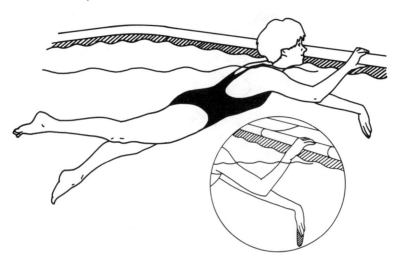

6. Advanced Soccer Kicks

Body parts strengthened: front of lower leg (tibialis anterior, extensor digitorum longus, extensor hallucis longus); front of thigh (quadriceps); back of thigh (hamstrings).

Put swim fins on both feet. Sit on the edge of the pool with your legs dangling in the water. Slowly kick one leg and then the other. As your foot nears the water surface, flex your ankle, raising the fin toward the surface. As you near the pool bottom, extend your foot, pointing the fin toward the bottom. One kick of each leg equals one repetition.

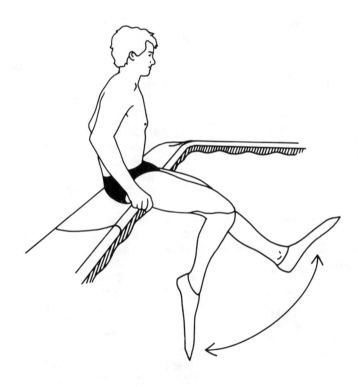

Contact Exercises

As your injury heals, you can continue the previous exercises and add these weight-bearing movements.

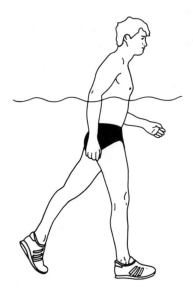

7. Water Walking

Body parts strengthened: front of thigh (quadriceps); back of thigh (hamstrings); calf (gastrocnemius, soleus, tibialis posterior, flexor hallucis longus, flexor digitorum longus); buttocks (gluteus maximus); hip (iliopsoas, sartorius, tensor fascia lata).

Stand in chest-deep water. Slowly walk from one side of the pool to the other. One step with each leg equals one repetition.

Note: You may want to wear shoes while walking. It will increase the support for your injury and reduce the impact with the pool bottom.

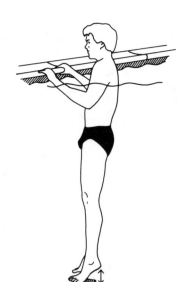

8. Double-Leg Heel Raises

Body parts strengthened: foot (intrinsic plantar flexors); calf (gastrocnemius, soleus, tibialis posterior, flexor hallucis longus, flexor digitorum longus).

Stand in chest-deep water, facing the pool edge, and hold the side of the pool. Slowly raise and lower your heels, keeping your body upright. Each double-leg heel raise equals one repetition.

9. Single-Leg Heel Raises
Body parts strengthened: foot (intrinsic plantar flexors); calf (gastrocnemius, soleus, tibialis posterior, flexor hallucis longus, flexor digitorum longus).

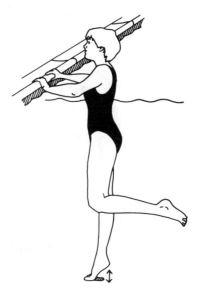

Stand in chest-deep water, facing the pool edge, and hold the side of the pool. Stand on your right leg. Slowly raise and lower your heel. One single-leg heel raise equals one repetition. Ten with the right leg followed by ten with the left is one set.

10. Single-Leg Hopping
Body parts strengthened: foot (intrinsic plantar flexors); calf (gastrocnemius, soleus, tibialis posterior, flexor hallucis longus, flexor digitorum longus); front of thigh (quadriceps); back of thigh (hamstrings).

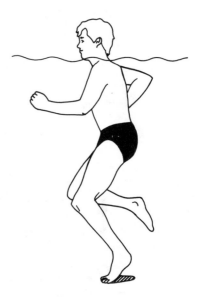

Stand on your left leg in neck- or chest-deep water. Hop from one side of the pool to the other. One hop equals one repetition. Do ten on the left and then ten on the right to complete one set.

FOOT, ANKLE, AND LOWER LEG WORKOUT

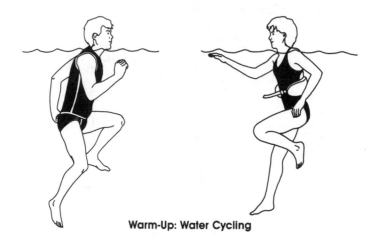

Warm-Up: Water Cycling

NONCONTACT EXERCISES

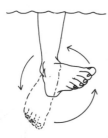

1. Foot Circles

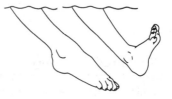

2. Ankle Flexions and Extensions

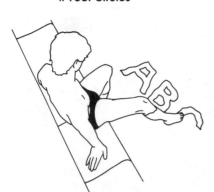

3. Alphabet

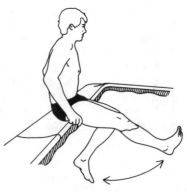

4. Soccer Kicks

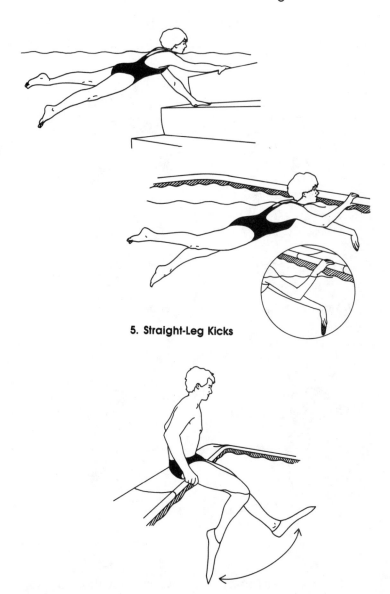

5. Straight-Leg Kicks

6. Advanced Soccer Kicks

CONTACT EXERCISES

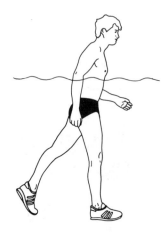

7. Water Walking

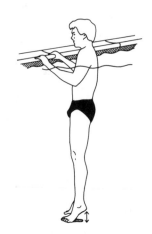

8. Double-Leg Heel Raises

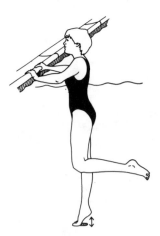

9. Single-Leg Heel Raises

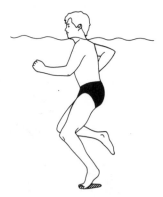

10. Single-Leg Hopping

WORKOUT SCHEDULE

Weeks 1 and 2

Frequency: Do the exercises three days a week with at least one rest day between training sessions.

Intensity: Do water warm-up and the first three exercises in this chapter.

Duration: Do two sets of 10 repetitions for each exercise.

Weeks 3 and 4

Frequency: Do the exercises five days a week with two rest days. Don't take two rest days in a row.

Intensity: Do water warm-up. In addition to the three exercises you did in weeks 1 and 2, add two exercises each week to the program.

Duration: Do three sets of 10 repetitions for each exercise.

Weeks 5 to 8

Frequency: Do the exercises six days a week. Take one rest day.

Intensity: Do water warm-up. In addition to the exercises you did in week 4, add one or two exercises each week until you are doing all the movements shown in this chapter.

Duration: Do four sets of 10 repetitions for each exercise.

6
Knees

The knee is a well-designed hinge joint, bending back and forth at the point where the tibia and fibula, two bones in the lower leg, meet the large femur in the thigh. If all we asked of our knee was to do its hinge motion in a gentle fashion for all of our lives, it would give us few problems. But we don't. Our knees are slammed from the side by a football tackle or ice hockey check, pounded and repeatedly bent and straightened as we run, and forced into a maximum flexed position as we slide into third base. No wonder the knee has a reputation as the most injured joint in the body. In almost all sports, the knee tops the list for the number of disabling injuries—the sort of injuries that keep you on the sidelines.

A look at the complexity of the knee joint will help you understand why so many things can go wrong when this joint is abused. The three large bones of the knee are strapped together by a system of tough ligaments, connective tissue that joins bone to bone. The largest and most prominent of these ligaments are on each side of your knee, and they are called the lateral (outer) and medial (inner) collateral ligaments. These tough structures help keep your knee from moving too far in a side-to-side motion. The anterior and posterior cruciate ligaments stabilize your knee front and back. Each connects with opposite sides of the tibia and femur, and they cross inside your knee, just about at the center of the joint.

The bones of the knee are cushioned by cartilage, pads of connective tissue located between the bones and lining the back of the kneecap. The sports pages always seem to have a report about one athlete or another with a torn knee cartilage. In most cases, the cartilage involved is either the medial or lateral meniscus, two pads located between the bones. It's the menisci that act as shock absorbers for the wear and tear of sports activity, and all too often the abuse they take causes them to tear.

The quadriceps tendon crosses the front of the knee, joining the muscles of the thigh to the kneecap. The bottom of the kneecap, or patella, is joined to the tibia bone in the lower leg by the patellar tendon. The kneecap is a sesamoid bone, which means it is not attached to any other bones in the body. It sits inside the quadriceps tendon, and this unusual location allows the kneecap to play an important role in the knee's remarkable mechanical engineering.

The kneecap protects the interior of the joint, acting like a shield against all the bumps and bruises we endure through life. Its most important job, however, is to increase the angle of the quadriceps tendon, and in doing this it increases the amount of force exerted by the thigh muscles on the joint. When you extend your leg to kick a soccer ball, the muscular contraction of the quadriceps muscles travels from the thigh, along the quadriceps tendon, to the kneecap and on to the tibia.

The kneecap, by increasing the angle of this pulley system, helps make your kick more powerful.

The movements of this hinge are controlled by muscles that are called knee extensors and knee flexors. You flex your knee when you bend it, such as when you sit in a chair or squat down. Your hamstrings, the large group of muscles on the back of your thigh, are principally responsible for knee flexion. Knee extension occurs when you straighten your leg, such as when kicking a soccer ball or jumping up to spike a volleyball. The quadriceps muscles on the front of the thigh are the knee extensors.

WATER EXERCISE AND YOUR KNEES

The most important thing to remember about the knee—especially when you are considering a water rehabilitation program—is that it is a weight-bearing joint, and not a very well protected one. Unlike the hip or shoulder joints, which are surrounded by muscles and tendons that help hold them in place, the bones and connective tissues of the knee are the first line of defense against the wear and tear of sport. When these parts of the knee are injured, weight-bearing movements are usually painful and you'll want to avoid them. This is why a knee injury can cause so much atrophy in the thigh muscles. It just hurts too much to put the joint through any amount of extension or flexion.

Water exercise, because it is non–weight bearing, is much more easily tolerated. The buoyancy of the water takes the stress off the joint and lets you strengthen your hamstring and quadriceps muscles. This, in turn, will add to the stability of the joint because the tendons of these muscles join them to the bones of the knee. The stronger your knee flexor and extensor muscles become, the less chance there is of reinjury to your knee joint, and the less wear and tear there will be on the nonmuscular parts of the joint. In fact, many knee injuries can be avoided if the hamstring and quadriceps muscles of the thigh are strong.

COMMON KNEE INJURIES

The one thing all the following injuries have in common is that they will make it difficult and often impossible to continue with your sport until the problem is corrected. This usually means you will need to take a break from your sport, a break that may mean several weeks off. The pool exercises in this chapter have been designed to help you recover from these common knee injuries.

Chondromalacia

The cartilage that lines the back of the patella can become irritated or actually worn away in some places because of overuse of the knee joint. This injury is common among runners. When you flex and extend your knee, the patella slides over a groove on the femur. When the patellar cartilage is damaged, the cushion between these two bones is diminished, causing pain and inflammation in the joint.

Patellar Tendinitis (Jumper's Knee)

This injury, as the name implies, is well known to long jumpers, triple jumpers and high jumpers. The repeated explosive jumping causes inflammation and small tears in the patellar tendon, usually just below the kneecap. Basketball and volleyball players also endure this injury, which will not heal unless the jumping activity is stopped until the pain is eliminated.

Medial Collateral Ligament Strain or Tear

You will recall that there are two large ligaments on the sides of the knee that help stabilize the joint. When the knee receives a blow on the outside of the joint, forcing the leg inward toward the body, fibers of the medial collateral ligament (on the inner side of your leg and knee) can be stretched or torn. This injury, which can require surgery, should be examined by a competent sports medicine physician. The lateral collateral ligament (on the outer side of your leg and knee) is seldom injured during sports because blows to the inside of the knee are rare.

Medial Meniscus Tear

The medial meniscus attaches to your medial collateral ligament. When a blow occurs on the outside of the leg—during a football or rugby tackle, for example— and is of sufficient impact to tear the medial collateral ligament, the medial meniscus may also tear. Surgery may be required to correct the problem.

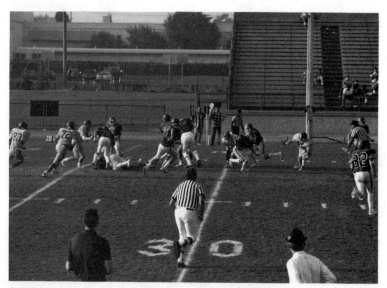

A severe blow to the knee during a football tackle can tear both the medial collateral ligament and the medial meniscus, which attaches to the ligament.

Chronic Overuse Injuries

Repeated bending and straightening of the knee joint can cause minute tears and inflammation in any one of the ligaments, tendons, or menisci. Runners, cyclists, rowers, and downhill and cross-country skiers are examples of athletes who put so much stress on the connective and cushioning mechanisms of the knee that this overuse syndrome develops. In particular, the two menisci are prone to developing small tears. The irritation in the joint may actually be caused by microscopic pieces of the cartilage that have worn loose and lodged somewhere in the joint. Persistent knee pain should be examined by a sports medicine physician. Usually you will need to stop your sport for a few weeks, during which time you can maintain your strength by doing the pool exercises that do not cause you pain.

Anterior Cruciate Ligament Tear or Strain

This may be the most audible injury in sport. If you have ever been unlucky enough to be near an athlete who tears his or her anterior cruciate—or worse, suffered this injury yourself—you will remember the loud "pop" that occurred as the ligament tore. The tear usually happens when you cut or twist sharply in a new direction or suddenly slow down, especially if you reduce speed by extending your leg in front of you. It can also happen if you receive a blow to the back of your leg. This may force the femur into the ligament, causing it to tear. See a physician if this injury occurs. Surgery may be necessary, followed by extensive rehabilitation. These pool exercises are a good starting point.

Posterior Cruciate Ligament Strain or Tear

This is not a common sports injury, but it can occur if the knee is hit from the front and severe hyperextension occurs. For example, it can happen when a football player is tackled at or below the knee when his feet are on the ground. Surgery may or may not be necessary, so see a physician. An extensive rehabilitation program may make surgery unnecessary, and these water exercises are a good starting point.

Dislocated Kneecap

Remember the kneecap sits inside the quadriceps tendon. If the quadriceps muscles contract forcefully while the leg is turned slightly inward and the knee is flexed (during a baseball swing, for example), the patella can be pulled off track. The damage that occurs to the surrounding structures and the tendon may require surgery and a lengthy rehabilitation, especially strengthening of the quadriceps muscles.

Iliotibial Band Tendinitis

This long band of connective tissue begins in your outer thigh, just below your hip, and continues down the outside of your leg, crossing the knee and inserting into the tibia bone in your shin. Repeated flexion and extension of the leg, common in sports such as running, rowing, skiing, and cycling, can cause irritation in this band as it rubs back and forth across a bony point on your femur called the lateral (on the outer side of your leg) epicondyle. The inflammation won't go away until you cut down on your training load. Your water recovery program should begin with the straight-leg exercises included in this section.

THE EXERCISES

Never do exercises that cause pain in the joint, especially at the site of your injury. Follow the workout guidelines presented in chapter 4.

Warm-Up
Water Cycling, as described on page 35.

1. Straight-Leg Walking
Body parts strengthened: all major muscles of the leg, including the front of the thigh (quadriceps); back of the thigh (hamstrings); calf (gastrocnemius, soleus, tibialis posterior, flexor hallucis longus, flexor digitorum longus); hip (ilipsoas, sartorius, tensor fascia lata).

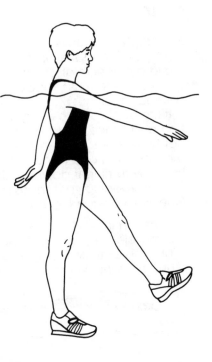

Stand in chest-deep water. Keeping arms and legs straight, walk from one side of the pool to the other. Don't bend your knees. One step with each leg equals one repetition.

Note: You may find it more comfortable to wear athletic shoes. They will let you grip the pool bottom and will absorb some of the impact of your walking.

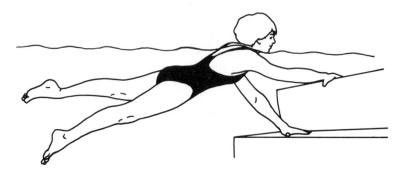

2. Straight-Leg Kicks

Body parts strengthened: hip (iliopsoas, sartorius, tensor fascia lata); inner thigh (adductor longus, brevis, and magnus; gracilis; pectineus); back of thigh (hamstrings); buttocks (gluteus maximus).

If the pool you are using has steps, float in the prone position and place your hands on the steps. If your pool does not have steps, float in the prone position, grip the side of the pool with one hand, and brace yourself with the other hand by turning it downward, as shown. *Kick your legs from the hip, keeping your knees straight.* Alternate left and right. One kick of each leg equals one repetition.

Note: An injury to the knee may weaken all the leg and hip muscles, especially if the pain makes you "favor" the injury. This exercise lets you keep your leg, hip, and buttocks muscles strong, without putting stress on your injured knee.

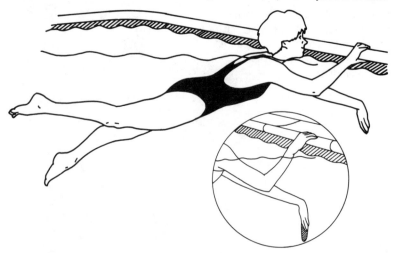

3. Leg Curls

Body parts strengthened:
back of thigh (hamstrings);
front of thigh (quadriceps);
hip (iliopsoas, sartorius, tensor
fascia lata).

Stand in chest-deep water,
holding the side of the pool,
with your right side next to the
pool edge. Bend your left leg
at the knee and then return it
to the starting position. One
curl equals one repetition. After ten repetitions, turn
around so your left side is next
to the pool edge and repeat
with the right leg. This is one
set.

Note: The leg you are exercising and the resting leg
should stay parallel through
the exercise. Don't allow the
working leg to move forward
or drift to the side. Avoid hyperextension of your lower
back by keeping your but-
tocks tucked.

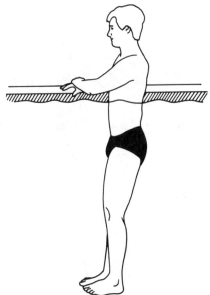

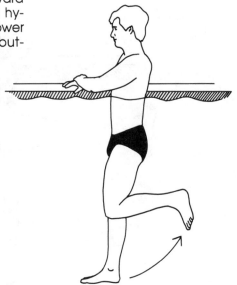

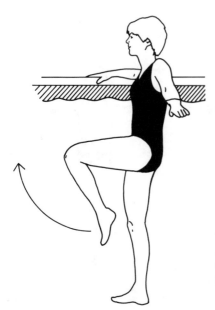

4. Knee Extensions

Body parts strengthened: front of thigh (quadriceps).

Stand in chest-deep water, holding the side of the pool, with your right side next to the pool edge. Raise your left leg with the knee bent. Straighten the leg by raising your lower leg in front of you. Return to the bent-knee position, keeping the thigh up. One raising and lowering of the lower leg equals one repetition. After ten repetitions, turn around so your left side is next to the pool edge and repeat with your right leg. This equals one set.

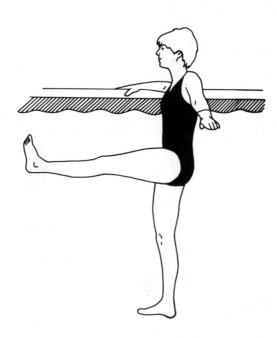

5. Gentle Knee Kicks

Body parts strengthened: front of thigh (quadriceps); back of thigh (hamstrings).

If your pool has stairs, float in the prone position with your hands resting on the steps. If your pool does not have steps, float in the prone position while holding a kick board in front of you. Gently kick the water by bending your knees. One kick of each leg equals one repetition.

Precaution: This is an excellent exercise for strengthening the quadriceps, but will aggravate your knee injury if done too vigorously. *Don't kick forcefully as this will cause your knee joint to hyperextend. Do the down stroke in a slow, controlled manner. Don't snap the knee joint.*

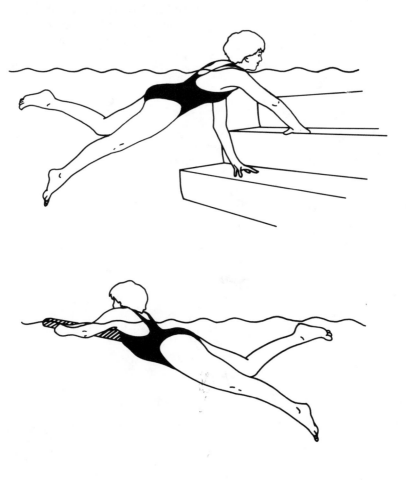

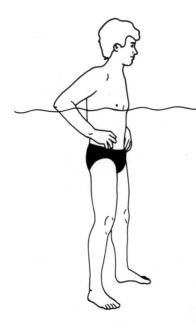

6. Squats
Body parts strengthened: front of thigh (quadriceps); back of thigh (hamstrings); buttocks (gluteus maximus).

Stand in chest-deep water with your hands on your hips. Keeping your feet flat on the bottom of the pool and your back straight, slowly bend your knees and then straighten your legs. Do not bend your knees beyond a 90-degree angle, which is the point at which your thighs are parallel to the bottom of the pool. One squat equals one repetition.

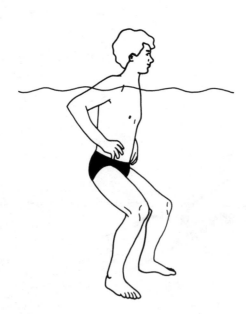

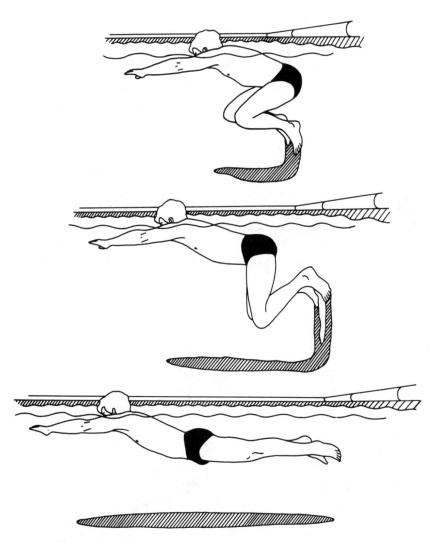

7. Wall Push-Offs

Body parts strengthened: front of thigh (quadriceps); back of thigh (hamstrings); buttocks (gluteus maximus).

Stand with your back next to the pool wall. Bend your knees and lift your feet against the wall. Gently push off away from the wall. One push-off equals one repetition.

Precaution: Do not do this vigorously as it may cause hyperextension of the knee.

8. Side Leg Raises

Body parts strengthened: hip (tensor fascia lata, iliopsoas, sartorius); inner thigh (adductor brevis, longus, and magnus; gracilus; pectineus); buttocks (gluteus medius and maximus); back of thigh (hamstrings).

Stand in chest-deep water, holding the side of the pool with your right side next to the pool edge. Slowly raise your left leg out to the side of your body. *Keep your toes facing straight ahead, not turned up toward the surface of the water.* Bring leg down to the starting position. Work against the resistance of the water as you move the leg in both directions. Each time you raise and lower your leg you have done one repetition. Complete ten repetitions; then turn around and repeat with right leg. This equals one set.

Precaution: Side-to-side movements with the leg can be painful to an injured knee. It is for this reason that we have put lateral leg lifts toward the end of the knee exercises. If this exercise causes you pain, wait until you are stronger before trying it again.

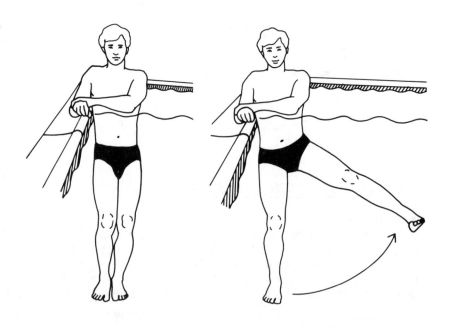

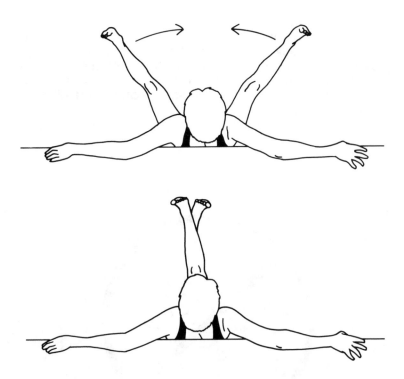

9. Scissors

Body parts strengthened: hip (tensor fascia lata, iliopsoas, sartorius); inner thigh (adductor brevis, longus, and magnus; gracilus; pectineus); buttocks (gluteus medius and maximus); back of thigh (hamstrings).

Stand in chest-deep water with your back against the pool wall. Grip the sides of the pool with your arms and hands. Bending at the hip, raise both legs straight up in front of you. Keep your buttocks and back against the pool wall. Spread your legs apart and bring them back together, crossing your feet at the ankles. Each time you bring your legs apart and together again, you have done one repetition.

Precaution: Side-to-side movements with the leg can be painful to an injured knee. It is for this reason that we have put scissors at the end of our knee workout. If this exercise causes you pain, wait until you are stronger before trying it again.

No Frog Kicking
The knee is a hinge joint. It is perfectly designed to move forward and back. Sideways motion with the leg may aggravate knee injuries, particularly a medial or lateral collateral ligament strain or tear. In particular, the frog-kick movement should *not* be part of your water rehabilitation program.

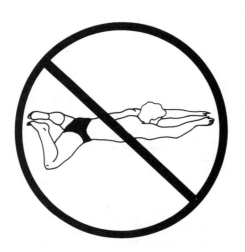

KNEE WORKOUT

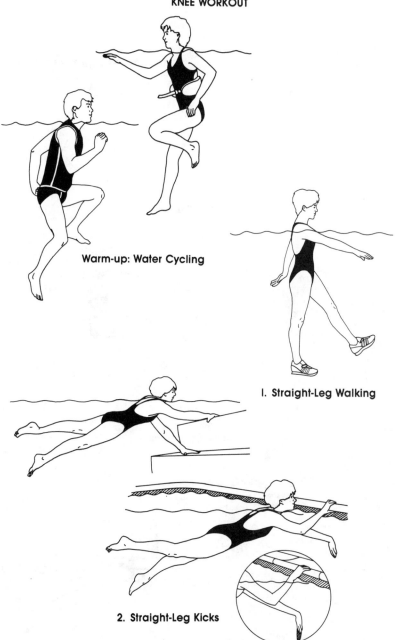

Warm-up: Water Cycling

I. Straight-Leg Walking

2. Straight-Leg Kicks

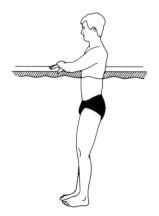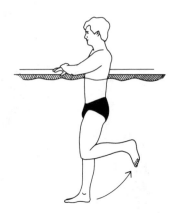

3. Leg Curls

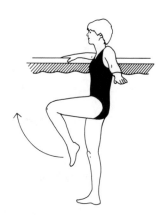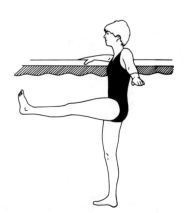

4. Knee Extensions

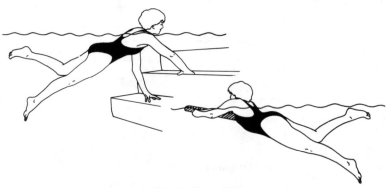

5. Gentle Knee Kicks

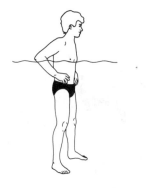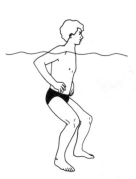

6. Squats

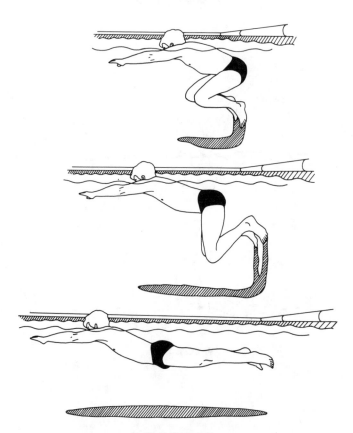

7. Wall Push-Offs

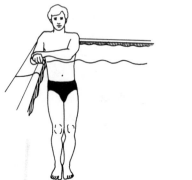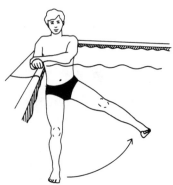

8. Side Leg Raises

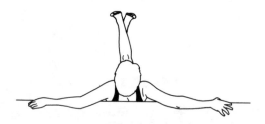

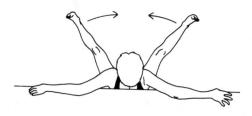

9. Scissors

WORKOUT SCHEDULE

Weeks 1 and 2

Frequency: Do the exercises three days a week with at least one rest day between training sessions.

Intensity: Do water warm-up and the first three exercises in this chapter.

Duration: Do two sets of 10 repetitions for each exercise.

Weeks 3 and 4

Frequency: Do the exercises five days a week with two rest days. Don't take two rest days in a row.

Intensity: Do water warm-up. In addition to the three exercises you did in weeks 1 and 2, add two exercises each week to the program.

Duration: Do three sets of 10 repetitions for each exercise.

Weeks 5 to 8

Frequency: Do the exercises six days a week. Take one rest day.

Intensity: Do water warm-up. In addition to the exercises you did in week 4, add one or two exercises each week until you are doing all the movements shown in this chapter.

Duration: Do four sets of 10 repetitions for each exercise.

7
Hips, Thighs, and Buttocks

One look at the anatomy of the hip joint and you'll know why injuries to this solid structure are so rare. The femur, the large thigh bone, has a round knob on the end. This knob fits snugly into a socket created by your pelvic bones, forming a very stable ball-and-socket joint. It's not the joint that will give you trouble, but rather the many muscles that are responsible for moving the ball and the socket and, therefore, the legs and hips. When these muscles are out of balance, overworked, or asked to move in a way they were not designed to move, they may become strained or torn.

Some of the best-known muscles in sport are in the thigh, namely the hamstring group on the back of the thigh and the four quadriceps muscles on the front of the thigh. The hamstrings are responsible for extending your hip, which is what you do when you lift your leg behind your buttocks. The quadriceps help flex your hip, or bring it forward, but their primary function is to straighten, or extend, the knee joint. As you can probably guess, these two muscle groups work together when you're playing your sport, and it is this relationship that causes some of the injuries. An imbalance in the strength of either of these muscle groups can lead to problems. If the quadriceps are stronger than the hamstrings, you may injure the muscles on the back of your thigh. If the hamstrings are stronger than the quadriceps, you may injure the muscles on the front of the thigh.

The inner thigh muscles attach to the lower part of the pelvis, and their job is to adduct your hip. (Adduction simply means moving toward the midline of the body. When you stand and swing one leg in front of the other, you're doing hip adduction.) These muscles on the inside of your thigh are called the adductor longus, adductor brevis, adductor magnus, pectineus, and gracilis. When someone has a pulled groin muscle, it's one of these muscles that's been injured.

The hip flexors, muscles on the front of your hip that attach to the pelvis and femur, work with the adductors and hamstrings to raise your leg in front of you. These muscles, the iliopsoas, tensor fascia lata, and sartorius, are powerful and extremely well developed in track and field athletes, especially jumpers.

The buttocks muscles round out this very powerful area of the body. The gluteus maximus, the largest and most prominent of this group, extends the hip. The primary job of its smaller cousins, the gluteus medius and minimus, is to lift the leg to the side and away from the body (this is called abduction), but they also assist the gluteus maximus in its job. Sprinters refer to this gluteal group as their "power pack." The strength of these muscles helps a sprinter power out of the blocks and achieve maximum flexion and extension of the hip joint, which translates into long, powerful strides. The hip rotators, small muscles buried deep below the larger gluteal muscles, turn your hip joint outward and assist in raising your leg behind you. When a soccer player moves in on the ball and turns his leg to kick with the side of his foot, these tiny hip rotators are what help move him into position.

YOUR WATER EXERCISE PROGRAM

We put considerable stress on the muscles of the hip and buttocks when we take part in sports. Imagine the power a weight lifter demands when he performs a squat with 300 pounds. How many times does a basketball or volleyball player jump during a game? Each time, the thigh and buttocks muscles put out a huge effort. A sprinter blasting out of the blocks forces the hip to move from maximum flexion to near maximum extension within a split second of the sound of the starter's gun.

When these muscles hurt, you have to give them time to heal before you get back in action. The thigh and buttocks muscles are often reinjured, mainly because the athlete puts stress on the injured area before it has recovered from the initial strain or tear. On the other hand, it is unrealistic to avoid using these muscles for several weeks. They will atrophy and weaken, which won't help your athletic performance and can lead to more problems.

These water exercises offer an answer to this dilemma. You can strengthen your muscles—provided the movement is pain free—without putting undue stress on the injured area. Your body is supported by the water, so your muscles do not have to work as hard to keep your body upright. More importantly, your legs are supported as you do the movements. You can move slowly; this permits you to work painlessly against the resistance of the water through the entire range of motion of the hip joint. And you'll be able to get started with your rehabilitation a lot sooner in the pool. Weight-bearing exercises on land are often painful, awkward, and difficult after you've suffered one of the injuries listed below.

HIP, THIGH, AND BUTTOCKS INJURIES

The pool exercises in this chapter have been designed to help you recover from these common hip, thigh, and buttocks injuries. The movements are geared specifically to strengthen muscles that are weakened by these injuries.

Hamstring Strain or Tear

This injury is common in football and in track and field, and it can be painfully dramatic when it occurs. The athlete, running full out, suddenly leaps into the air, grasping the back of the thigh. A moment later the dejected athlete is writhing on the ground, the victim of a torn hamstring. The fibers of one of the hamstring muscles may have been weak or partially torn when the race started, but leaning forward, putting the hip into maximum extension, pushed the muscle over the edge. A long-distance runner, on the other hand, may feel a nagging ache in the back of the thigh for a couple of weeks. This slow-onset hamstring pull may take a while to reach its painful peak, but eventually it can become as disabling as a sudden injury.

This is one of those injuries that you've got to take your time rehabilitating. Running on land too soon will reinjure the muscle fibers. You'll reduce the risk of a reoccurrence if you begin your running and strengthening program in the pool where movements are non-weight bearing.

Quadricep Contusion (Charley Horse)

In contrast to its funny name, this is one of the most serious leg injuries in sports. It usually occurs in football, rugby, or hockey when the player is struck by equipment or another player. The blow causes the blood vessels and/or quadriceps muscle fibers to be crushed and, as you can imagine, a large, painful bruise results. If it is not rehabilitated correctly, including strengthening exercises for the hamstring and quadriceps muscles, there can be a reduction in the range of motion of the knee joint. Once the injured area is no longer painful—which can take several weeks if proper emergency care is not administered when the injury occurs—you can begin to strengthen the thigh muscles, which will have been weakened by the inactivity and damage caused by the blow. The non-weight-bearing exercises in the pool will be much more tolerable, especially in the early weeks of recovery.

Stress Fracture of the Femur

This is a rare but serious injury. The large muscles that surround this bone usually protect it from the shock of repeated impact that occurs during downhill skiing or excessive long-distance running. But, when the impact is transferred to the bone, tiny fractures can occur on its surface. All activity should be non–weight bearing until the fractures have healed, making the pool the ideal environment for maintaining muscular strength and aerobic fitness during the weeks of recovery.

Quadriceps Strain or Tear

Muscle imbalance in which the hamstrings are stronger than the quadriceps can cause these muscles on the front of your thigh to strain or tear. A movement that may be possible for the hamstrings, such as explosive jumping or sprinting, puts the quadriceps in peril, and the muscle fibers give way. Strengthening this muscle group after the injury is a critical part of rehabilitation. You will be able to do the non-weight-bearing movements in the pool in the weeks you are working toward returning to your running program. The thigh is supported by the water, and movements are more likely to be pain free.

Adductor (Groin) Strain or Tear

Just about the only athletes with very strong inner thigh muscles are jockeys. The bent position of the hip, while using the legs to hold on to the horse, recruits these muscles for both of their jobs—pulling the legs toward the body and flexing the hip. The resulting adductor strength puts jockeys at low risk for this nagging injury. Athletes in other sports, especially running and soccer, are more likely to strain or tear these muscles, in some cases because the adductor group is not sufficiently warmed up before a race or game or because the group is not strong enough to perform on the same level as the hamstrings and quadriceps. A tear or strain in the adductor group can persist, and your return to dry-land training must be carefully timed or you risk reinjury. The pool exercises, particularly Side Leg Raises, Leg Circles, and Scissors, are excellent for strengthening injured groin muscles.

Outer Hip Pain

If you feel pain on your outer hip, you may have strained the tensor fascia lata muscle or the large tendon to which it attaches. This tendon, called the iliotibial band, stretches from the hip to the knee. This is a common running injury and usually means you need to strengthen all of the muscles of the thigh. In some cases, outer hip pain is an indication that you have a weakness in the lower back. Because the muscles in the buttocks and hip attach at the lower back, pain from lower back injury may show up on the outer hip. If the pain persists, you should see a physician to rule out any structural damage to the bones and discs in the spine. Whether your injury is in the back or in the actual hip area, water exercise is an excellent prescription. It will let you strengthen the muscles without putting weight on the injury.

Hip Pointer

This is an impact injury common in football. The iliac crest, a bony ridge that forms the upper edge of your pelvis, is bruised by contact with equipment or another player. Usually the bruise occurs at the most prominent point on the iliac crest, the protruding area toward the front of the pelvis just below your belt line. This painful injury often results in muscle spasms, which will make it difficult to return to your sport until the tenderness has subsided. You can maintain your leg and buttocks strength with the water exercises listed here, provided they do not cause you pain in your injured hip.

Piriformis Spasm

The piriformis is one of those little hip-rotator muscles found below the gluteals. Despite its small size, when the piriformis is in spasm, it can cause you to curtail most of your activity. You'll feel the pain in your buttocks, back, and sometimes down the outside of your leg. This last symptom is sciatica, or inflammation of the sciatic nerve, which begins at your lumbar spine and continues down your legs. A spasming piriformis can compress the sciatic nerve. Sciatica may be a symptom of a lower back injury, and you should see a physician if you experience radiating pain down your leg. If your injury is in fact a piriformis spasm, it is important to avoid weight-bearing activity until the spasm is eliminated, or you risk chronic sciatica. Water exercise will keep the muscles strong until the spasm subsides. The

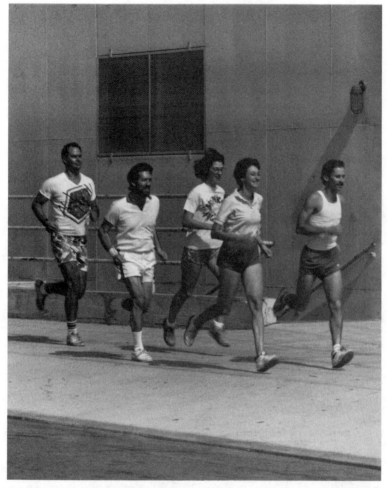

Excessive running, especially on pavement, can cause tearing and inflammation in the iliotibial band, a large tendon that stretches from your hip to your knee. Pool running and strengthening exercises will take the stress off the tendon until it heals.

piriformis goes into spasm because the other muscles of the hip are weak, requiring the buttocks muscle to put out more effort than it can handle. Strengthening your thigh and buttocks muscles—as the exercises in this chapter do—will help prevent a reoccurrence of the injury.

THE EXERCISES

Never do exercises that cause pain in the joint, especially at the site of your injury. Follow the workout guidelines presented in chapter 4.

Warm-Up
Water Cycling, as described on page 35.

I. Side Leg Raises
Body parts strengthened: outer thigh (tensor fascia lata); inner thigh (adductor brevis, longus, and magnus; gracilis; pectineus); hip (iliopsoas, sartorius); buttocks (gluteus medius and maximus); back of thigh (hamstrings).

Stand in chest-deep water, holding the side of the pool. Your right side should be next to the pool edge. Slowly raise your left leg out to the side of your body. *Keep your toes facing straight ahead, not turned up toward the surface of the water.* Bring the leg down to the starting position. Work against the resistance of the water as you move the leg in both directions. Each time you raise and lower your leg you have done one repetition. Complete ten repetitions; then turn around and repeat with right leg. This equals one set.

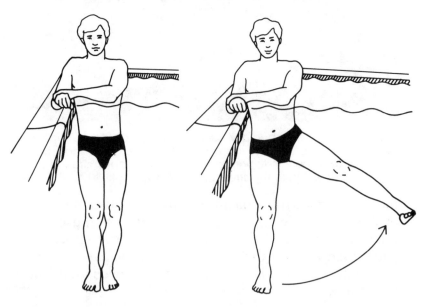

2. Straight-Leg Kicks

Body parts strengthened: hip (iliopsoas, sartorius); inner thigh (adductor longus, brevis, and magnus; gracilis, pectineus); back of thigh (hamstrings); outer thigh (tensor fascia lata); buttocks (gluteus maximus, medius, and minimus).

With your buttocks and back against the pool wall, hold the side of the pool with your arms and hands. Raise both legs to hip level. Kick your legs, keeping them straight and alternating left and right. Raise your legs to hip level with each kick. One kick of each leg equals one repetition.

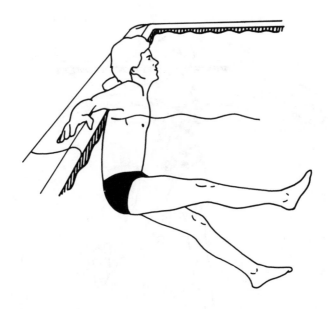

3. Leg Circles

Body parts strengthened: hip (iliopsoas, sartorius); inner thigh (adductor longus, brevis, and magnus; gracilis; pectineus); back of thigh (hamstrings); outer thigh (tensor fascia lata); buttocks (gluteus maximus, medius, and minimus).

Stand in chest-deep water with your right side next to the pool edge. Holding the side with your right hand for balance, raise the left foot slightly flexed, draw a circle, using the heel of your foot as the "pen." Each circle should be as large as you can make it without aggravating your injury. Work within your own range of motion. Do five circles clockwise, then five circles counterclockwise. Turn around and repeat with the right leg. This equals one set.

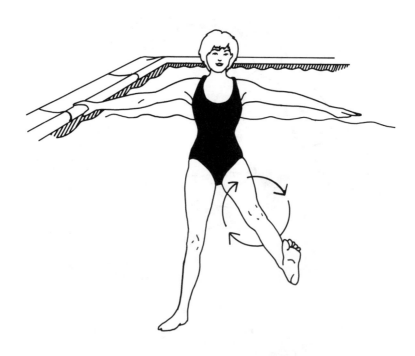

4. Leg Curls

Body parts strengthened:
back of thigh (hamstrings);
front of thigh (quadriceps);
hip (iliopsoas, sartorius, pectineus).

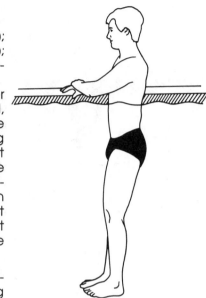

Stand in chest-deep water holding the side of the pool, with your right side next to the pool edge. Bend your left leg at the knee and then return it to the starting position. One curl equals one repetition. After ten repetitions, turn around so your left side is next to the pool edge and repeat with the right leg. This is one set.

Note: The leg you are exercising and the resting leg should stay parallel through the exercise. Don't allow the working leg to move forward or drift to the side. Avoid hyperextension of your lower back by keeping your buttocks tucked.

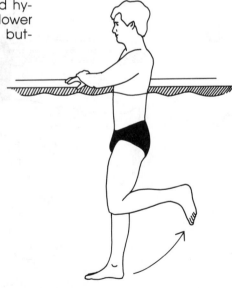

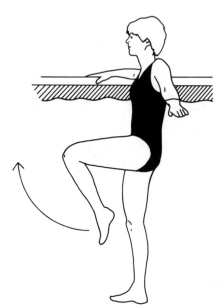

5. Knee Extensions

Body parts strengthened: front of thigh (quadriceps).

Stand in chest-deep water, holding the side of the pool, with your right side next to the pool edge. Raise your left leg with the knee bent. Straighten the leg by raising your lower leg in front of you. Return to the bent-knee position, keeping the thigh up. Raising and lowering of the lower leg once equals one repetition. Complete ten repetitions; then turn around so your left side is next to the pool edge and repeat with your right leg. This is one set.

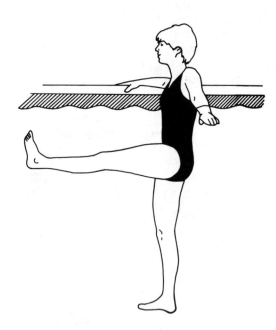

6. Straight-Leg Raises

Body parts strengthened: hip (iliopsoas, sartorius); front of thigh (quadriceps); inner thigh (adductor longus, brevis, and magnus; gracilis; pectineus); back of thigh (hamstrings); buttocks (gluteus maximus, medius, and minimus).

Stand in chest-deep water with your right side next to the pool edge. Hold the edge for balance. Slowly raise your left leg in front of you. Keep the leg straight. Return to the starting position. Raising and lowering your leg once equals one repetition. After ten repetitions, turn around and repeat with the right leg. This is one set.

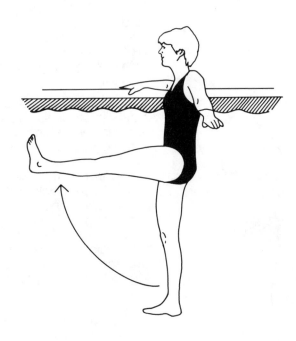

7. Hip Extensions

Body parts strengthened: hip (iliopsoas, tensor fascia lata); inner thigh (adductor longus, brevis, and magnus; gracilis; pectineus); back of thigh (hamstrings); buttocks (gluteus maximus, medius, and minimus).

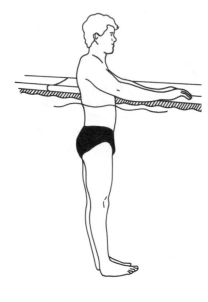

Stand in chest-deep water. Face the pool side and hold the edge for balance. Raise your left leg behind you. Keep the leg and back straight. Don't allow your lower back to arch. Each time you raise and lower your leg, you have done one repetition. Complete ten repetitions. Repeat with the right leg. This equals one set.

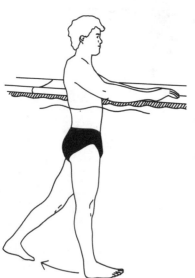

Note: Don't make a swayback in order to move your leg further behind you. This may aggravate your lower back and will not enhance the effect of the exercise. To protect your back and to get maximum benefit from this movement, lift your leg in a slow, controlled manner. Don't move quickly or try to use the momentum of your leg to lift your leg further behind you.

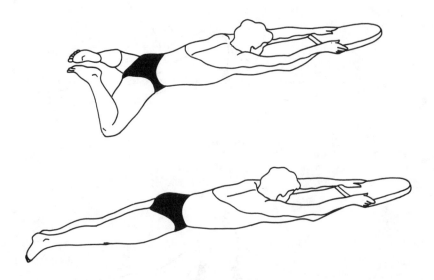

8. Frog Kicks

Body parts strengthened: inner thigh (adductor longus, brevis, and magnus; pectineus; gracilis); buttocks (gluteus maximus, medius, and minimus); hip (iliopsoas, tensor fascia lata, sartorius); back of thigh (hamstrings); front of thigh (quadriceps).

Hold a kick board in front of you as you float in the prone position. Keeping your legs together, bend your knees toward your body. Then straighten them to each side and squeeze your legs together. Each kick counts as one repetition.

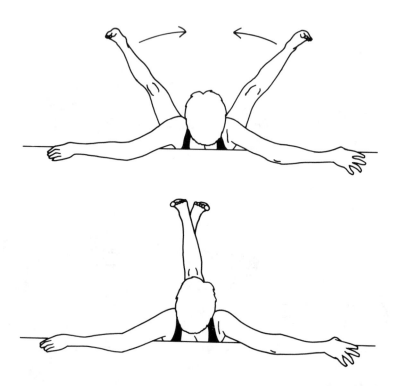

9. Scissors

Body parts strengthened: hip (tensor fascia lata, iliopsoas, sartorius); inner thigh (adductor brevis, longus, and magnus; gracilus; pectineus); buttocks (gluteus medius and maximus); back of thigh (hamstrings).

Stand in chest-deep water with back against pool wall. Grip the sides of the pool with your arms and hands. Raise both legs up in front of you, bending at the hip. Keep your buttocks and back against the pool wall. Spread your legs apart and bring them back together, crossing your feet at the ankles. Each time you bring your legs apart and together again you have done one repetition.

HIP, THIGH, AND BUTTOCKS WORKOUT

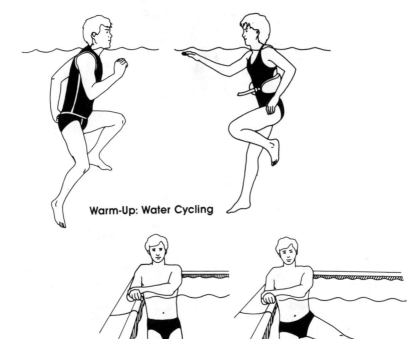

Warm-Up: Water Cycling

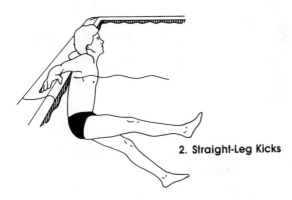

1. Side Leg Raises

2. Straight-Leg Kicks

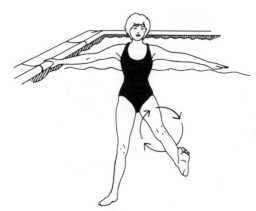

3. Leg Circles

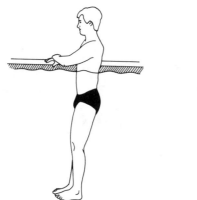

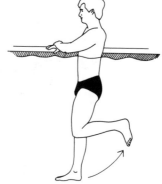

4. Leg Curls

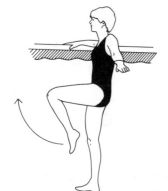

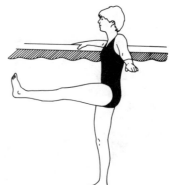

5. Knee Extensions

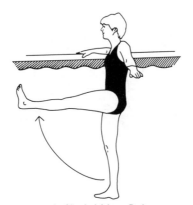

6. Straight-Leg Raises

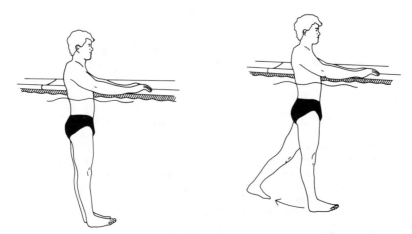

7. Hip Extensions

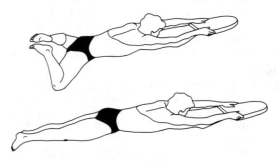

8. Frog Kicks

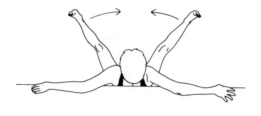

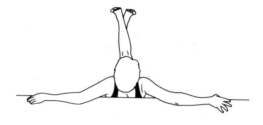

9. Scissors

WORKOUT SCHEDULE

Weeks 1 and 2

Frequency: Do the exercises three days a week with at least one rest day between training sessions.

Intensity: Do water warm-up and the first three exercises in this chapter.

Duration: Do two sets of 10 repetitions for each exercise.

Weeks 3 and 4

Frequency: Do the exercises five days a week with two rest days. Don't take two rest days in a row.

Intensity: Do water warm-up. In addition to the three exercises you did in weeks 1 and 2, add two exercises each week to the program.

Duration: Do three sets of 10 repetitions for each exercise.

Weeks 5 to 8

Frequency: Do the exercises six days a week. Take one rest day.

Intensity: Do water warm-up. In addition to the exercises you did in week 4, add one or two exercises each week until you are doing all the movements shown in this chapter.

Duration: Do four sets of 10 repetitions for each exercise.

8
The Back

Eighty percent of all Americans will experience back pain during their lives. Athletes put extra demands on the spine and muscles of the back and are particularly prone to back pain. Gymnasts twist their backs into such incredible positions that you might think the back was made of rubber bands and Silly Putty®. Runners pound the pavement—and their backbones—as they log hundreds of miles a year. Football linemen drive their head and shoulders into the opposition, and it's the spine that takes the brunt of becoming a human battering ram.

The backbone is a marvelous assembly of thirty-three separate bones, and it can usually take whatever abuse you give. Strong but still very flexible, your spine can move in six directions: forward and back, side to side, and rotating to the left and right. The vertebrae, those twenty-four rounded bones in the spine, become larger as they descend, because of the increased weight these bones must carry. The smaller vertebrae in the neck bear the weight of our head, while the large vertebrae in the lower back must support half our body weight.

The vertebral column, although it is continuous, is divided into three distinct sections. The neck consists of seven bones which are called the cervical vertebrae. Just below the neck bones are the twelve thoracic vertebrae. Ten of your ribs attach to these vertebrae to form the thoracic cavity, a cage that protects your heart and lungs. The five lumbar vertebrae are the bones in the small of your back, just below the thoracic vertebrae. The sacrum, five fused bones that form a triangular shape, and the coccyx (or tailbone), composed of four small bones, complete the spine.

The vertebrae aren't just stacked up like white chips on a poker table but are carefully padded and protected by resilient discs that sit between them. The outside of these intervertebral discs is a tough fibrous tissue that forms a casing around the soft, gel-like substance inside. Acting like tiny cushions between the vertebrae, the discs absorb the forces that twist, turn, and bend the back.

Each individual vertebra has bony processes that protrude out to the rear and to the sides. (A *process* is the medical term for something that juts out or protrudes, like the stick on the bottom of a Popsicle.) The muscles of the back attach to these protruding sections and can move the spine in all of its many directions. Together, the vertebrae form a canal that extends from the brain to the pelvis, protecting the spinal cord. They also provide a passageway for the major nerves of the arms and legs, which is why an injury to the vertebrae can cause pain in your arms or legs.

CHECK YOUR POSTURE

A healthy back has a natural curve. If you were to look at the spinal column from the side, this curve would look like the letter S. If you stand with your chest for-

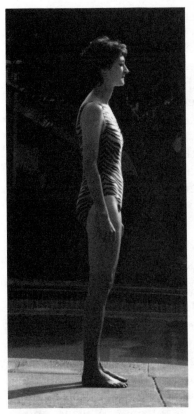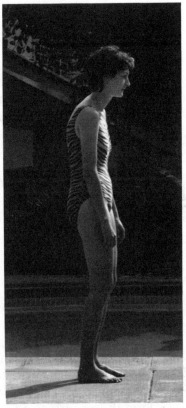

Standing with your chest forward, shoulders back, and head over the spine maintains the healthy S shape of the spinal column.

A head-forward, round-shouldered posture changes the curve of the spine to an unhealthy C shape, putting stress on the muscles, joints, and intervertebral discs.

ward, your shoulders back, and the head over the spine, you maintain the healthy S shape of the spinal column. But too often human endeavor doesn't do much for our posture. Working behind a desk can be worse for your back than many sports. Everyday activities such as driving and watching TV can be harmful as well. When the head is pitched forward, the round-shouldered position changes the curve of the spine. It flattens the lower back and flexes the thoracic and cervical spine. This posture turns your spine from an S shape into a C shape, putting far more stress on the muscles, joints, and intervertebral discs.

A majority of all back problems would be alleviated if correct posture was maintained. In particular, keeping your head over your shoulders, instead of jutting out in front of you, greatly reduces the strain on the back muscles and bones. The farther forward your head is placed, the greater the length of the lever arm between your spine and your head—and the more stress you are putting on your cervical vertebrae. You can't change the weight of your head, but you can eliminate this lever arm by bringing your neck and head back over your body.

Once you have your head over your neck, it is easier to keep your chest forward and your shoulders back. This puts the curve back in your lumbar spine—and your entire back into its healthy S shape again. And this means your muscles and bones are not subjected to undue stress.

Maintaining good posture requires strong back and abdominal muscles. The back muscles, because they are always used to hold us upright, are usually much stronger than your abdominal muscles. A weak abdomen can wreak havoc on your posture. Think of your trunk muscles as a girdle. For the entire girdle to provide support, it must be tight all around. If the front part of the girdle is weak, you will sag in that direction. This is exactly what happens if your abdominal muscles are weak. The abdomen sags forward, exaggerating the curve of the lumbar spine, which in turn leads to back pain. We once treated one of the top Dodgers players who was complaining of back pain. The Dodger trainers checked him out and discovered that even though he was extremely fit, he couldn't do five sit-ups. Abdominal strengthening just hadn't been part of his training program. The trainers put him on a program to strengthen his abdominals and after several weeks, he could do 300 sit-ups and his back pain had disappeared.

WATER EXERCISE AND YOUR BACK

Water exercise is excellent for your back. In the water the force of gravity is about one-tenth that on land. The stress of your body weight on your spine is considerably reduced. At the same time, your back and abdominal muscles are constantly working to stabilize your trunk in the water. This makes the "girdle" that surrounds your spine much stronger.

The exercises in this chapter are specifically designed to strengthen the muscles of your back and abdomen. Again, strengthening these muscles will help you maintain a healthy posture, which in turn will reduce your back pain.

COMMON BACK INJURIES

The exercises in this chapter will help you recover from these common back injuries and will strengthen muscles weakened by these injuries.

Muscle Spasm

This may be the most common back complaint. It occurs when you twist or bend your back—often when lifting. Suddenly your back seizes up. The pain can be anywhere in the back, but the most frequent location is across the lower back just above the buttocks. The muscles tighten up painfully, and it is difficult to move. It may feel as if your back is "locked" or as if it "catches" when you try to move in one direction. You have strained one of the back muscles, and it has gone into a painful spasm. The spasm should subside—and pain will be eliminated—after three or four days. Repeated episodes of back spasming may indicate your abdominal or back muscles are weak or that you have an injury to a disc or spinal bone.

These water exercises are a safe way to begin to strengthen the muscles, providing the movements are pain free. If your pain persists for more than a week, especially if you have pain radiating down your legs and arms, see a physician.

Disc Bulge

This injury usually occurs when you are lifting a heavy object and you suddenly twist. Doing a dead lift or squat with poor technique—such as leaning forward or twisting while holding the weight—is a common cause of injury to the intervertebral discs. When there is a bulge in the disc, the tough cartilage that surrounds the gel-like substance actually bulges out of position, placing pressure on the nerves that pass through the vertebra. The nerve becomes irritated, and you feel pain along the nerve pathway.

If the bulge occurs in the lumbar spine, the most common site, the pain will be in the buttocks, radiating down your leg as it follows the sciatic nerve. In some cases, the pain may be in the back only. If the bulge is in the cervical spine, you will feel pain in your shoulder and arm as it follows the path of the pinched cervical nerve. See a physician if you have these symptoms. (These injuries rarely happen in the thoracic spine because these vertebrae are attached to the ribs and have a limited range of motion.)

Because your body weight is supported by the water, water exercise reduces the compression that gravity places on the disc.

Herniated Disc

The symptoms of a herniated disc are similar to those of disc bulge, except that numbness and loss of reflex in

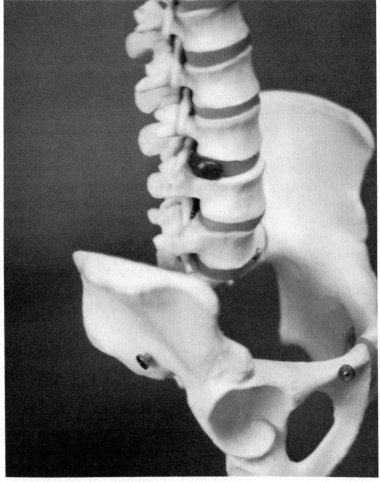

The lighter gray areas between the vertebrae are the interverte-bral discs. These discs act as shock absorbers for the bones of the spine. The darker spot in the center of the photograph indicates a disc that has herniated.

the arm or leg may also be present. A herniation means that disc cartilage has actually torn, allowing the interior gel-like substance to flow out of the disc and impinge on the nerve. Though not common, the herniated disc is a serious injury. If you have any of the symptoms of a bulge or herniation, get to a physician as soon as possible.

Some disc herniations will repair themselves without surgery if you have a proper program of stretching and strengthening under the care of a physical therapist. The water exercises here will take the compression off the spine and allow you to strengthen your abdominal and back muscles, important steps in alleviating the symptoms of a bulge or herniation.

Spondylolysis

This is a stress fracture of the vertebra caused by a wearing down of the bone. This injury can happen in sports in which high-impact landings are common, such as gymnastics, pole vaulting, long and triple jump, and diving. Minute cracks form in the vertebra, which can turn into complete fractures if the stress continues. You will feel pain at the site of the stress. A water exercise program will let you strengthen your back and abdominal muscles and take the stress off the bone while it heals.

Spondylolisthesis

This injury plagues two divergent groups of athletes—gymnasts and football linemen. It occurs with excessive and repeated bending of the spine—such as that experienced by a gymnast practicing a routine, or a lineman blocking an opposing player and forcing his own spine backward into hyperextension. It is also a further progression of spondylolysis. Continued stress causes the small bones on the sides of the vertebra to break, and the vertebra moves forward of the others. Spondylolisthesis usually occurs in the lumbar spine. You will feel pain in the immediate area, and it may radiate down the left or right side of the buttock and into the leg. In rare cases, surgery may be necessary. Water exercise will reduce the stress on the bone while it heals and will strengthen the trunk muscles, reducing or eliminating symptoms.

THE EXERCISES

Never do exercises that cause pain in the joint, especially at the site of your injury. Follow the workout guidelines presented in chapter 4.

Warm-Up
Water Cycling, as described on page 35.

I. Water Walking
Body parts strengthened:
back (erector spinae); abdomen (rectus abdominis); front of thigh (quadriceps); back of thigh (hamstrings); calf (gastrocnemius, soleus, tibialis posterior, flexor hallucis longus, flexor digitorum longus); buttocks (gluteus maximus); hip (iliopsoas, sartorius, tensor fascia lata).

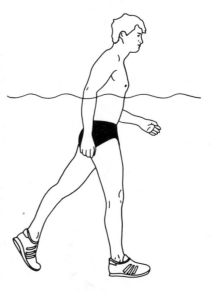

Stand in chest-deep water. Slowly walk from one side of the pool to the other. One step with each foot equals one repetition.

Note: You may want to wear shoes while walking. It will increase the support for your injury and reduce the impact with the pool bottom.

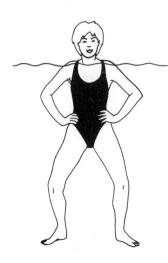

2. Trunk Twists with Hands on Waist

Body parts strengthened: abdomen (external and internal obliques); back (erector spinae).

Stand in shoulder-deep water with legs apart at shoulder width and feet flat on the pool bottom. Place hands on hips and bend knees slightly. Slowly turn to the right as far as possible and then to the left as far as possible. Return to the front position. This completes one repetition. Move only your upper body and keep your feet in place on the pool bottom. Avoid hyperextension of the lower back by tucking your buttocks.

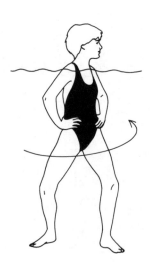 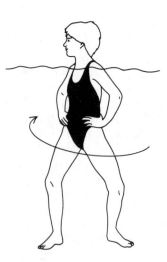

3. Trunk Twists with Arms Extended

Body parts strengthened: abdomen (external and internal obliques); back (erector spinae).

Stand in shoulder-deep water with legs apart at shoulder width and knees slightly bent. Extend arms straight out to the sides, parallel to the surface of the water. Keep palms down. Slowly turn your body to the right as far as possible and then to the left as far as possible. Return to the front position. This completes one repetition. Move only your upper body and keep your feet in place on the pool bottom. Keep your arms under water throughout the movement.

Note: You may increase resistance by turning your hands so they are at right angles to the pool bottom, as shown in the top-left illustration.

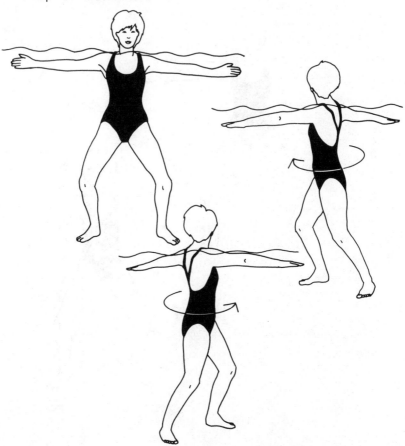

4. Arm Fanning
Body parts strengthened: back (erector spinae); abdomen (internal and external obliques, rectus abdominis); shoulder (latissimus dorsi, teres major and minor, anterior and posterior deltoid, subscapularis); chest (pectoralis major).

Stand in shoulder-deep water with legs apart at shoulder width and knees slightly bent. With hands open and palms forward, place arms straight out to the sides, parallel to the surface of the water. Bring your arms together, keeping them straight and parallel to the surface. Return to the starting position, pulling arms away from the midline of the body. This completes one repetition.

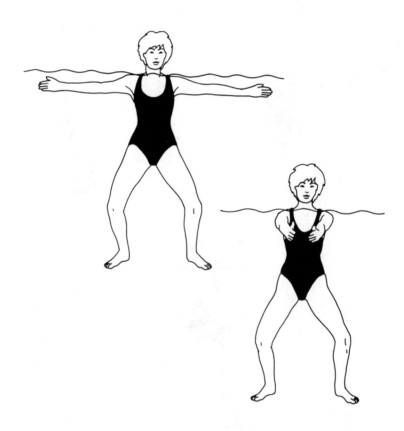

5. Digging

Body parts strengthened: back (erector spinae); abdomen (rectus abdominis); chest (pectoralis major); shoulder (latissimus dorsi, posterior and anterior deltoid, teres major); arm (biceps, triceps).

Stand in shoulder-deep water with legs apart at shoulder width and knees slightly bent. Extend arms straight out in front, parallel to the surface of the water, and cup your hands with the palms turned downward. Slowly push down, moving the arms past the body and behind your torso. Turn your hands so palms are again downward and pull arms back to starting position. This completes one repetition. Keep your arms underwater throughout the movement.

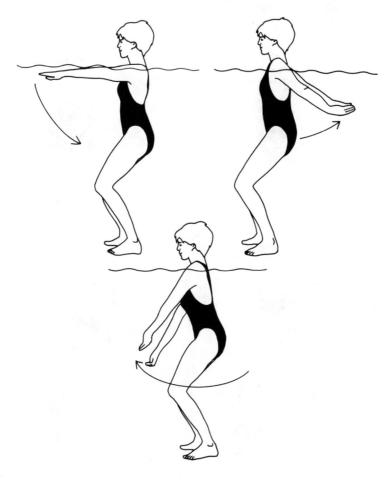

6. Arm Crossing

Body parts strengthened: back (erector spinae, trapezius, rhomboids); abdomen (rectus abdominis, internal and external obliques); chest (pectoralis major and minor); shoulder (latissimus dorsi, deltoid, and supraspinatus).

Stand in shoulder-deep water with legs apart at shoulder width and knees slightly bent. Begin with arms parallel to the surface of the water and straight out to the side. With hands cupped and palms downward, swing arms down in front of the body and then return to the parallel position. Swing arms down behind the body and then return to the parallel position. This completes one repetition. To reduce strain on lower back, keep buttocks tucked. Arms remain underwater throughout the movement.

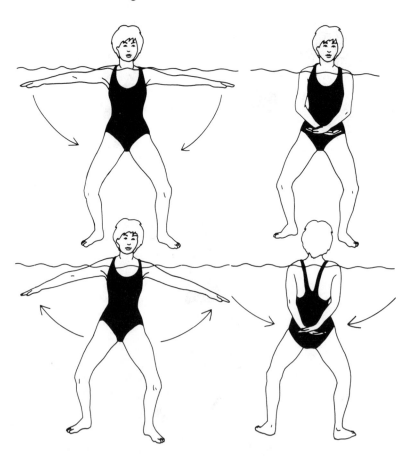

7. Knee Lifts

Body parts strengthened: abdomen (rectus abdominis, internal and external obliques); hip (iliopsoas, sartorius, tensor fascia lata); back (erector spinae); buttocks (gluteus maximus).

Hang by your arms from the side of the pool. Your feet should not touch the pool bottom. Keeping your buttocks against the pool wall, extend your legs straight below you. Bend knees to chest. Return to starting position, legs extended straight toward bottom. One lift and return equals one repetition.

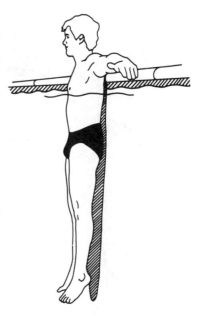

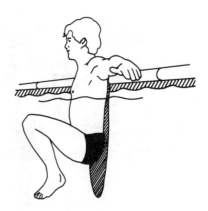

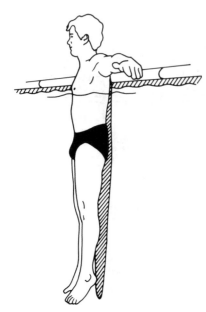

8. On-the-Wall Leg Raises

Body parts strengthened: abdomen (rectus abdominis, external and internal obliques); back (erector spinae); hip (iliopsoas, tensor fascia lata, sartorious); buttocks (gluteus maximus).

Hang by your arms from the side of the pool. The water must be deep enough that your feet do not touch bottom. Keep your buttocks against the wall. Begin with your legs extended straight below you. Slowly raise both legs to the surface, keeping them straight and together. Return to the starting position. This equals one repetition.

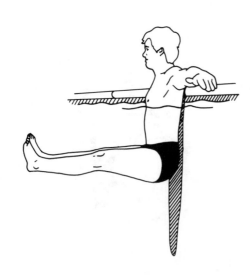

9. Wall Sit-Ups

Body parts strengthened: abdomen (rectus abdominis, external and internal obliques).

Rest calves on the pool deck and float on your back in the pool. Cross your arms on your chest. Gently curl upward so your shoulders just break the surface of the water. Hold for a count of ten and return to starting position. This equals one repetition.

Note: Do not hold your breath. Gently breathe in and out as you count to ten.

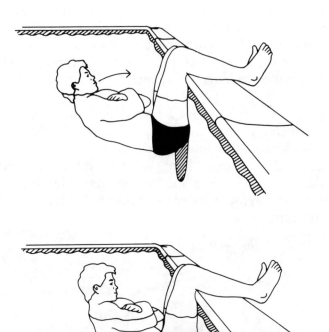

SWIMMING

Swimming is one of the best exercises for your back. The muscles of your abdomen and back work to keep your body on top of the water as you swim. The stress of gravity on your back is eliminated because your body weight is suspended in the water. We have recommended swimming only for back injuries. You may not know how to swim, or you may have poor swimming technique. Many athletes who take part in sports do not enjoy swimming. If, however, you have a back injury and you know how to swim, a few minutes of swimming, in addition to the water exercises presented in this chapter, will greatly relieve your pain and will speed your recovery. If you do not know how to swim, do not attempt to learn these strokes when you are injured.

Begin with strokes that let you float on your back. These are easy on the spinal column. The freestyle tends to extend your lower back, which can aggravate an injury. If you have them, wear a waterskiing belt, snorkle, and mask when you do the freestyle. Never do the breaststroke, which puts considerable stress on the lumbar spine.

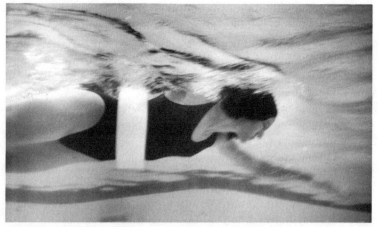

Wearing the waterskiing belt makes the freestyle much easier for less proficient swimmers.

Elementary Backstroke

If you have ever taken swimming lessons, even beginner's level, you can probably do the elementary backstroke. The arm motion works all of the major muscles of the back, and your abdominal muscles are working to keep your body parallel to the surface. It's the perfect stroke to begin with if you want to include a few laps of swimming after you finish up your water exercise program. Continue for up to ten minutes, but not to the point of muscular fatigue or pain.

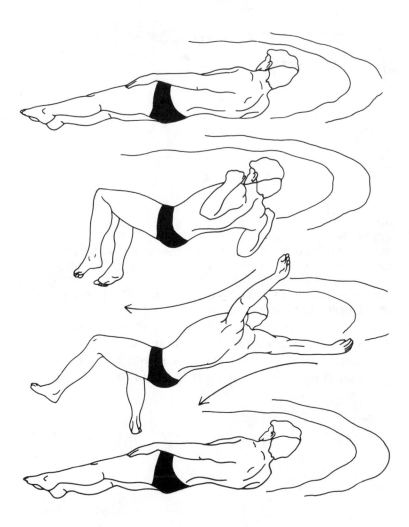

Backstroke

If you already enjoy swimming, you probably feel comfortable doing the backstroke. It works your back and abdominal muscles. If you find the elementary backstroke too slow or awkward, try the backstroke for a while. Do your lap swimming after you do the water exercises. Continue for up to ten minutes, but not the point of muscle fatigue or pain.

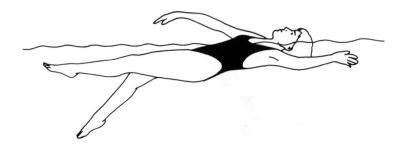

Freestyle

Swimming facedown tends to accentuate the curve in your lower back, which is why we recommend the strokes in which you are floating on your back. But, swimming the freestyle—or "front crawl"—is perfectly safe if you follow a few simple guidelines:

1. Wear a snorkel and mask when you swim. You will be able to keep your spinal column straight, rather than constantly rotating it to breathe.

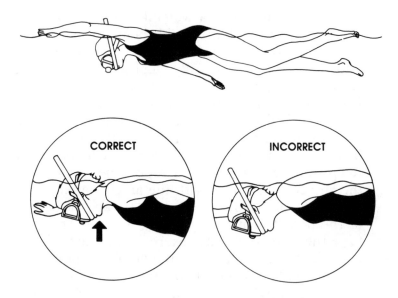

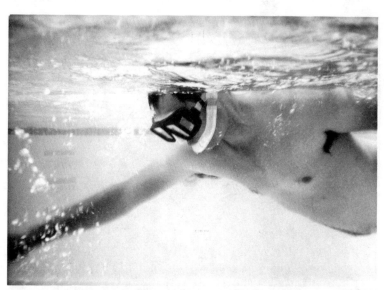

Turning your head to breathe while swimming may aggravate your back injury. A snorkel and mask allow you to breathe without rotating your spine.

2. If you have one, wear a waterskiing belt. For extra support, wear it with the buckle behind you. The belt will support your lower back and increase your buoyancy. This is especially helpful if you are not a strong swimmer.

3. If you do not have a waterskiing belt, keep your abdomen tucked when you swim and do not let your back sag toward the bottom of the pool. See the full-body illustration on page 123 for correct alignment.

4. Keep your head in line with your spine, as shown in the circled illustration with the arrow on page 123. Do not let your neck and head sag toward the bottom of the pool. Swim for up to ten minutes after you have finished your water exercise program. If your back hurts, especially in the lumbar spine, stop swimming. You will probably find it a lot easier and enjoyable to swim on your back, especially if you do not have a belt to help support your lower back.

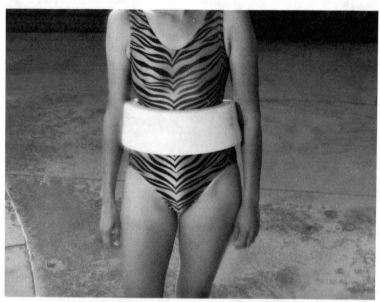

When doing the freestyle, wear a waterskiing belt with the buckle at the back. This will help support your lower back.

BACK WORKOUT

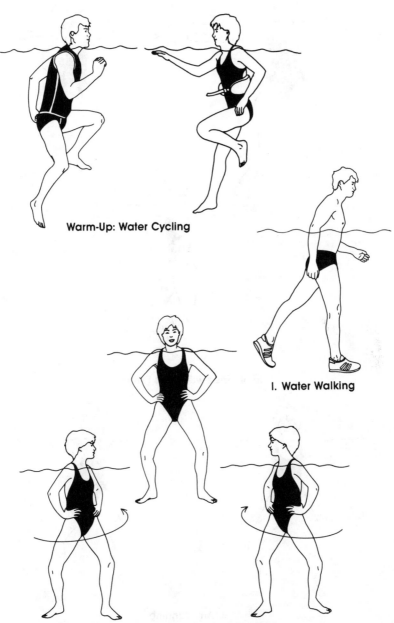

Warm-Up: Water Cycling

1. Water Walking

2. Trunk Twists with Hands on Waist

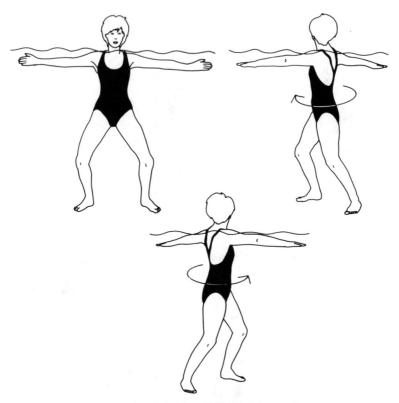

3. Trunk Twists with Arms Extended

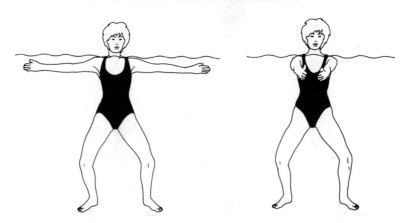

4. Arm Fanning

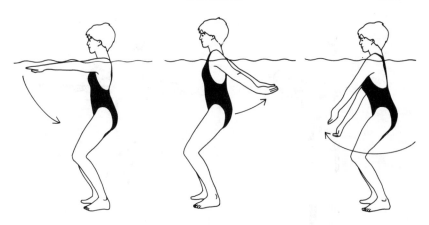

5. Digging

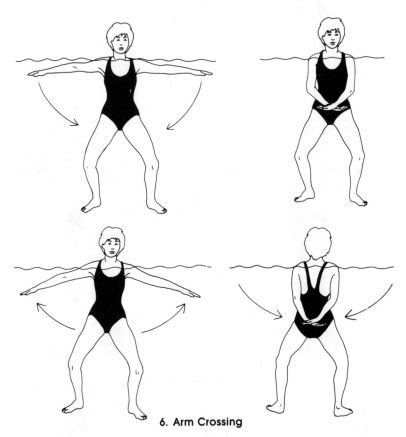

6. Arm Crossing

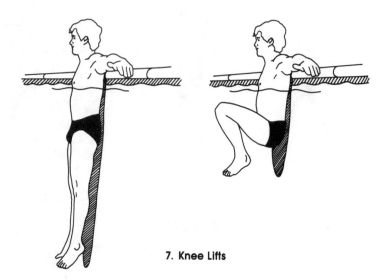

7. Knee Lifts

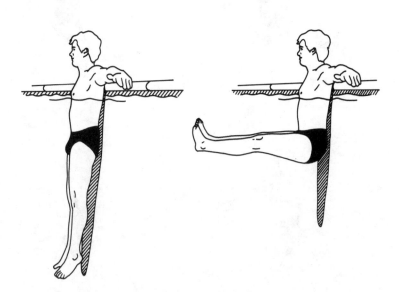

8. On-the-Wall Leg Raises

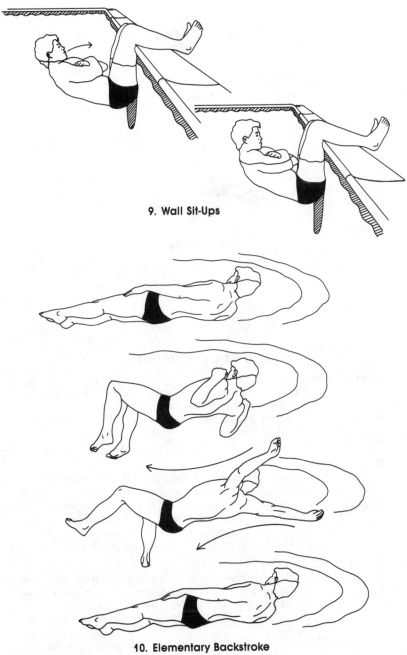

9. Wall Sit-Ups

10. Elementary Backstroke

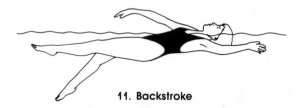

11. Backstroke

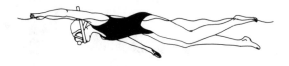

12. Freestyle

WORKOUT SCHEDULE

Weeks 1 and 2
Frequency: Do the exercises three days a week with at least one rest day between training sessions.

Intensity: Do water warm-up and the first three exercises in this chapter.

Duration: Do two sets of 10 repetitions for each exercise.

Weeks 3 and 4
Frequency: Do the exercises five days a week with two rest days. Don't take two rest days in a row.

Intensity: Do water warm-up. In addition to the three exercises you did in weeks 1 and 2, add two exercises each week to the program.

Duration: Do three sets of 10 repetitions for each exercise.

Weeks 5 to 8
Frequency: Do the exercises six days a week. Take one rest day.

Intensity: Do water warm-up. In addition to the exercises you did in week 4, add one or two exercises each week until you are doing all the movements shown in this chapter.

Duration: Do four sets of 10 repetitions for each exercise.

9
Shoulders

The shoulder has more mobility than any other joint in the body. Its remarkable flexibility allows major league pitchers to throw ninety-mile-per-hour strikes and outfielders to reach up and catch high fly balls. The shoulder can maintain this flexibility only if its complex physiology is in proper working order. When any part of the system is injured, mobility is decreased and you'll feel pain. Since we use our shoulder for so many movements—from tying our shoes to throwing a javelin—a loss of shoulder range of motion is usually very debilitating.

The shoulder's unique design gives it the flexibility on which we depend. The bones of the shoulder are the scapula, or shoulder blade, the clavicle, or collarbone, and the humerus, the bone of your upper arm. Together they form a shallow ball-and-socket joint. In fact, the socket is so shallow that the bones would not hold together if they were not surrounded by an extensive system of ligaments, tendons, and muscles, all of which work together to keep the bones in place.

The muscles and tendons closest to the ball and socket joint, deep within the shoulder, are called the rotator cuff. The four muscles of this cuff are the supraspinatus, infraspinatus, teres minor (on the back of the shoulder), and the subscapularis (on the front of the shoulder). Tendons linking these muscles to the bones of the shoulder are also part of this cuff, which, as its name implies, surrounds the joint and stabilizes the bones. It's your rotator cuff that keeps your humerus bone from slipping out of the shoulder socket.

A small ligament joins the clavicle to a bony point on the scapula called the acromion process. This junction is called the acromioclavicular joint, and it is highly vulnerable to injury in sports. You are asking a lot when you expect this tiny ligament to endure a football tackle or a slam into the boards during a hockey game. Sometimes the ligament just isn't strong enough to hold the bones in place, as you will see when we explain shoulder separation.

An injury to any part of the shoulder's support system will reduce the effectiveness of the joint. Strengthening the muscles that surround the bones of the shoulder joint is the most important thing you can do to speed your recovery from injury. You need strong muscles to stabilize the joint and allow the shoulder to move through its full range of motion.

WATER RECOVERY FOR YOUR SHOULDER

Shoulder injuries are so common among baseball pitchers that the trainers for the Los Angeles Dodgers take the preventive approach. They treat every pitcher as if he has a shoulder injury, whether he feels pain or not. Part of that treatment is to spend a certain amount of time in the pool doing strengthening exercises similar to the ones shown here. The trainers and players found, as will you, that the pool is an excellent place to strengthen a shoulder. The water supports your arms, taking most of the pull of gravity off the bones and soft tissues (ligaments, tendons, and muscles) around the joint. In this reduced-stress environment, you can move the shoulder slowly through its range of motion, using the resistance of the water to build strength.

You will notice that all of the exercises are done under the surface as you stand in shoulder-deep water. Your arms never come above shoulder level. There's a good reason for this. Raising your arm above your shoulder, whether to the side or to the front, is almost always painful if you have a shoulder injury. The water acts as a safeguard against this movement. If your arms are coming out of the water, you're probably lifting them too high and you may be aggravating your injury.

COMMON SHOULDER INJURIES

The exercises in this chapter are specifically designed to help you recover from these common shoulder injuries. The movements will strengthen muscles that are weakened by these injuries.

Rotator Cuff Tendinitis

This is an overuse injury that is common in sports that involve throwing. Swimmers and tennis players may also suffer from this painful inflammation of the tendons because of the repetitive overhead arm movements that these sports require. The tendons become inflamed due to overuse, and the muscles to which these tendons attach are weakened because of reduced mobility and pain.

Rotator Cuff Tear

This is one of those injuries that really hurts when you raise your arm over your head. A tendon in the rotator cuff develops small tears either from overuse or from a trauma such as a shoulder dislocation. Minor tears will usually heal after a brief withdrawal from the sport combined with a strengthening program for the rotator cuff muscles. Major tears severely limit shoulder mobility. These more serious tears are usually caused by trauma, such as a football tackle or falling off a horse, and require surgery.

Broken Collarbone (fractured clavicle)

There's a good reason rodeo cowboys and parachute jumpers roll when they land on the ground rather than stop their fall with outstretched arms. They know that landing on their hands is a sure way to break the clavicle bone. This fracture occurs when you extend your arms to break a fall and the force of the impact is transmitted up your arm to the clavicle.

Deltoid Tear or Strain

In contact sports, especially football and rugby, tackling can cause strains or tears of the tendons and muscle tissue of the deltoid, the muscle that caps your shoulder joint. Muscle weakness occurs because of the injured fibers.

Shoulder Separation

The ligament of the acromioclavicular joint, the point where the clavicle is joined to the scapula, can be torn or strained if you fall on the top of your shoulder or an outstretched hand. Wrestling, rugby, football, and especially ice hockey are the sorts of contact sports that put this joint at risk. Your shoulder is going to be in a sling for a while after this injury, so the muscles of your shoulder girdle will be weakened from inactivity. Once you have your doctor's okay to begin rehabilitation, it is important you work these muscles, bringing them up to the level of strength you had before the injury. These water exercises are a safe way to begin your rebuilding program.

Shoulder Dislocation

It's painful just to think about the trauma that occurs inside your shoulder when the humerus is pulled out of the socket. The ligaments, tendons, and muscles that surround the shoulder are pulled and torn to such a degree that this injury can cause permanent instability in the joint.

An anterior shoulder dislocation is the most common form of this injury. The arm is forced backward while the elbow is bent, something that might happen in a football or rugby tackle. The force is so great that the ligaments, tendons, and muscles surrounding the joint cannot hold the head of the humerus in place and it slips forward. Any number of these support structures may be torn—rotator cuff tears are common with a dislocation—and the head of the humerus may even fracture as it comes in contact with the acromion process on the scapula.

Because of all the muscles that cross the back of your shoulder, the posterior dislocation accounts for only about 2 percent of all dislocations, but it's just as serious and debilitating as the anterior variety. Again, it usually occurs during a tackling situation: the arm is forced into a flexed position, the support system gives way, and the humerus slips out the back of the socket.

Once your shoulder is put back in place—and this should be done immediately and *only* by a physician—it will be immobilized for several weeks, after which you must dedicate yourself to strengthening the muscles of the shoulder girdle. This is your main insurance against repeated dislocations. These water exercises have been used by many athletes with this injury, and they are an excellent starting point for your recovery.

THE EXERCISES

Never do exercises that cause pain in the joint, especially at the site of your injury. Follow the workout guidelines presented in chapter 4.

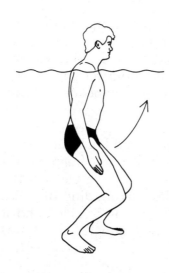

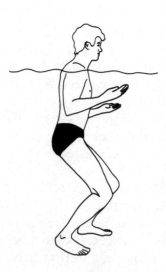

Warm-Up
Water Cycling or Water Jogging, as described on pages 35 and 36.

I. Double-Arm Pulls
Body parts strengthened: front of upper arm (biceps, brachialis).

Stand in shoulder-deep water with legs apart at shoulder width and knees slightly bent. Begin with arms straight down at your sides. With palms facing upward, raise both hands toward your body, bringing them as close to your upper body as you can without discomfort. Keep elbows and upper arms next to your sides. Relax and slowly lower forearms to the starting position. This completes one repetition.

Note: Strengthening your upper arm muscles, both front and back, is important if you have a shoulder injury. These muscles cross the shoulder joint, and if they are weak, you may experience shoulder pain. (The triceps, the muscle group at the back of the arm, is particularly neglected.) This exercise and the following, the Double Arm Pushes, are an excellent beginning for your shoulder rehabilitation because they strengthen the upper arm muscles and keep your shoulder strong. Because these exercises do not directly involve movement of the shoulder joint, they should cause no discomfort in your shoulder.

2. Double-Arm Pushes
Body parts strengthened: back of upper arm (triceps).

Stand in shoulder-deep water with legs apart at shoulder width and knees slightly bent. Bend elbows 90 degrees and turn palms toward the bottom of the pool. Keeping elbows and upper arms close to the sides of the body, push your hands down until they are at your sides. Relax and slowly raise forearms to the 90-degree starting position. This completes one repetition.

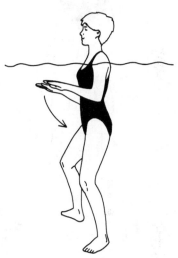

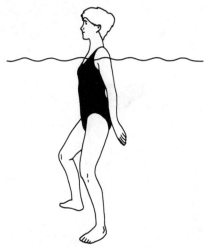

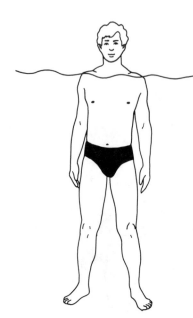

3. Straight-Arm Raises
Body parts strengthened:
shoulder (latissimus dorsi, deltoid, supraspinatus); back
(rhomboids); chest (pectoralis major and minor).

Stand in shoulder-deep water with legs apart at shoulder
width and knees slightly bent.
Begin with arms at your sides,
palms toward body. Raise
arms straight out to the sides,
to just below the surface, and
then lower them to your sides.
This completes one repetition.

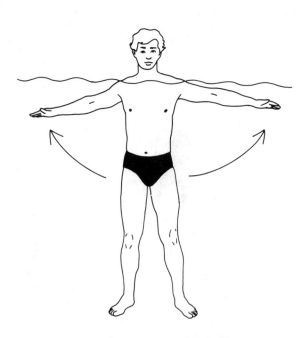

4. Thirty-Degree Arm Raises
Body parts strengthened:
shoulder (supraspinatus).

Stand in shoulder-deep water with arms at your sides. Keep your hand open, the back of your hand toward your body, and the little finger turned toward the pool surface. Raise your right arm at a 30-degree angle away from the body to just below the surface. Return to the starting position. This equals one repetition. Do ten with the right and ten with the left to complete one set.

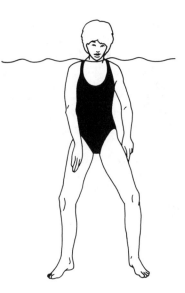

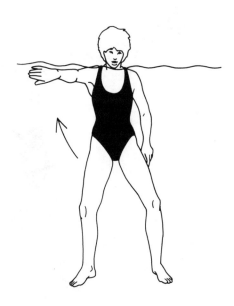

5. Arm Fanning

Body parts strengthened: back (erector spinae), abdomen (internal and external obliques, rectus abdominus); shoulder (latissimus dorsi, teres major and minor, anterior and posterior deltoid, subscapularis); chest (pectoralis major).

Stand in shoulder-deep water with legs apart at shoulder width and knees slightly bent. With hands open and palms forward, place arms straight out to the sides, parallel to the surface of the water. Bring your arms together, keeping them straight and parallel to the surface. Return to the starting position, pulling arms away from the midline of the body. This completes one repetition.

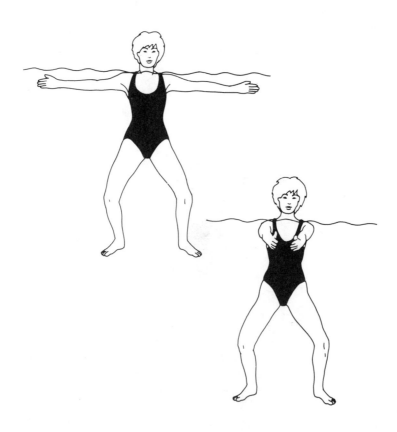

6. Arm Crossing

Body parts strengthened: back (erector spinae, trapezius, rhomboids); abdomen (rectus abdominus, internal and external obliques); chest (pectoralis major and minor); shoulder (latissimus dorsi, deltoid, and supraspinatus).

Stand in shoulder-deep water with legs apart at shoulder width and knees slightly bent. Begin with arms parallel to the surface of the water and straight out to the side. With hands cupped and palms downward, swing arms down in front of the body and return to the parallel position. Swing arms down behind the body and return to the parallel position. This completes one repetition. To reduce strain on the lower back, keep buttocks tucked.

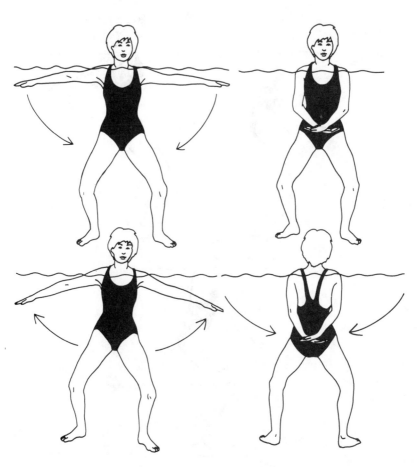

7. Digging

Body parts strengthened: back (erector spinae); abdomen
(internal and external obliques, rectus abdominis); shoulder
(latissimus dorsi, posterior and anterior deltoid, teres major);
arm (biceps, triceps).

Stand in shoulder-deep water with legs apart at shoulder
width and knees slightly bent. Extend arms straight out in
front, parallel to the surface of the water, and cup your
hands with the palms turned downward. Slowly push down,
moving the arms past the body and behind your torso. Turn
your hands so palms are again downward and pull arms
back to starting position. This completes one repetition.

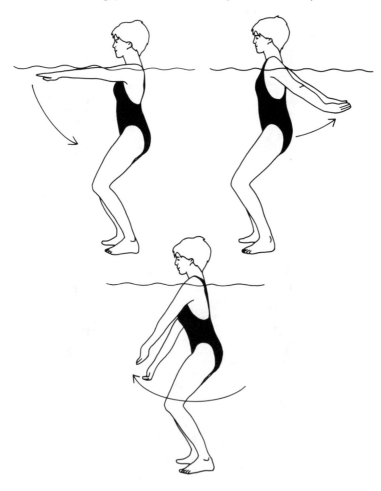

8. Arm Circles with Hands on Shoulders
Body parts strengthened: shoulder (anterior, middle, and posterior deltoid; teres major and minor; infraspinatus).

Stand in shoulder-deep water with your legs apart at shoulder width and knees slightly bent. Place hands on shoulders. Draw circles backward with your elbows. The circles should be as large as you can make them, without aggravating your injury. Work within your own range of motion. One circle equals one repetition.

Note: There is a good reason to do this exercise only toward the back. The shoulder muscles on the back of your body are usually much weaker than those on the chest and front of the shoulder. This muscle imbalance is one of the reason's for a "round-shouldered" appearance and may be the cause of your shoulder injury. Moving your arm backward strengthens the weak muscles and helps correct this imbalance.

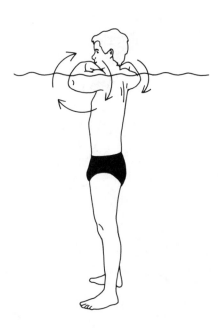

9. Straight-Arm Circles

Body parts strengthened: shoulder (anterior, middle, and posterior deltoid; teres major and minor; infraspinatus).

In shoulder-deep water, extend arms to the side of your body parallel to the surface. Draw circles backward with your arms. The circles should be as large as you can make them, without aggravating your injury. Work within your own range of motion. One circle equals one repetition.

Note: This exercise is done only toward the back for the same reasons described in the previous exercise.

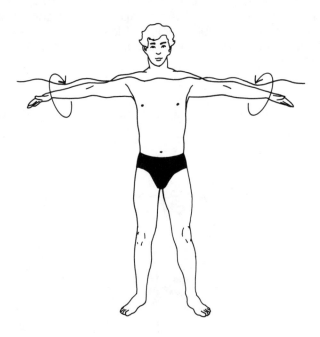

10. Bent-Elbow Arm Swings

Body parts strengthened: shoulder (teres minor, infraspinatus, anterior and posterior deltoid, subscapularis); back (latissimus dorsi).

Stand in shoulder-deep water with your left side next to the edge of the pool. Balance yourself with your left hand and arm. Tuck your right elbow into your ribs and bend it 90 degrees. Keeping your upper arm against the body, fan your forearm away from the body and then back across your abdomen. Each time you move your forearm away from your body and back to your abdomen you have done one repetition. Keep the hand open and perpendicular to the pool bottom with your thumb pointing toward the surface.

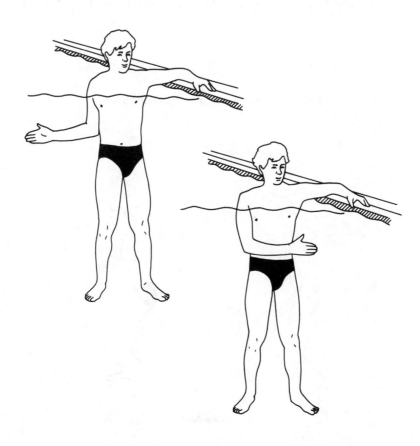

SHOULDER WORKOUT

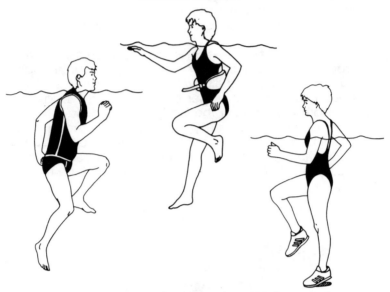

Warm-Up: Water Cycling or Water Jogging

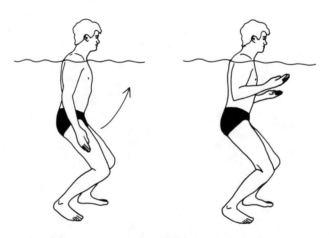

I. Double-Arm Pulls

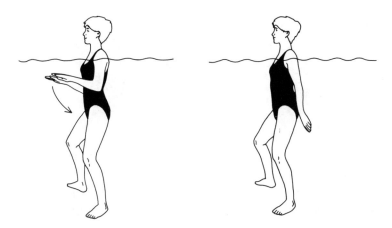

2. Double-Arm Pushes

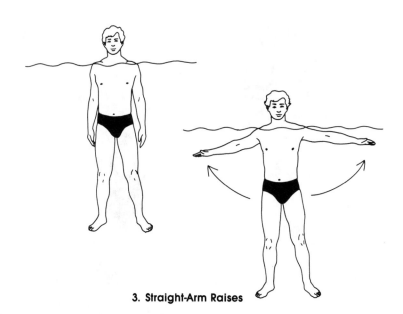

3. Straight-Arm Raises

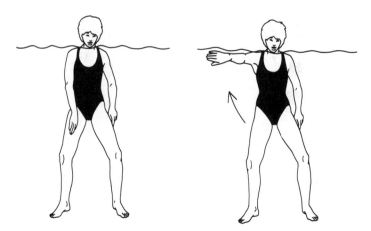

4. Thirty-Degree Arm Raises

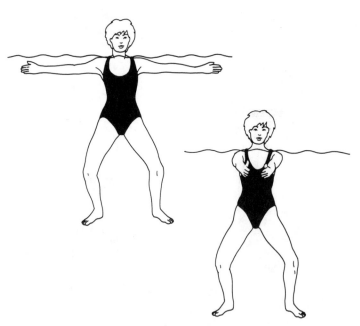

5. Arm Fanning

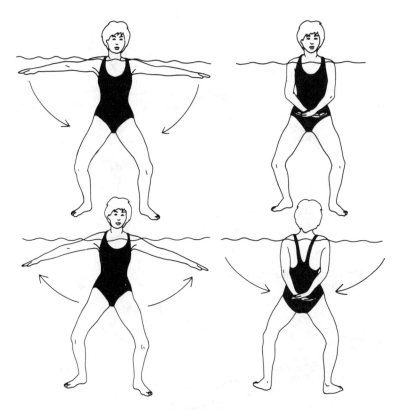

6. Arm Crossing

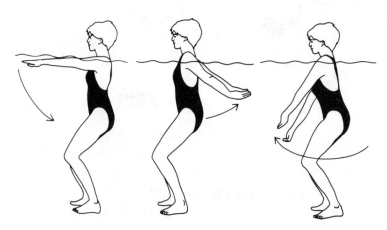

7. Digging

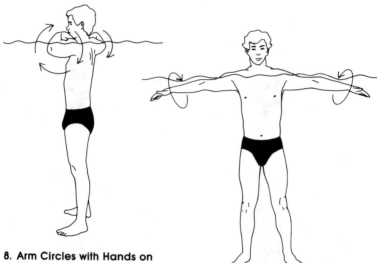

8. Arm Circles with Hands on Shoulders

9. Straight-Arm Circles

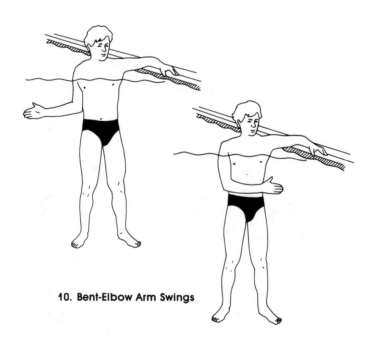

10. Bent-Elbow Arm Swings

WORKOUT SCHEDULE

Weeks 1 and 2
Frequency: Do the exercises three days a week with at least one rest day between training sessions.
Intensity: Do water warm-up and the first three exercises in this chapter.
Duration: Do two sets of 10 repetitions for each exercise.

Weeks 3 and 4
Frequency: Do the exercises five days a week with two rest days. Don't take two rest days in a row.
Intensity: Do water warm-up. In addition to the three exercises you did in weeks 1 and 2, add two exercises each week to the program.
Duration: Do three sets of 10 repetitions for each exercise.

Weeks 5 to 8
Frequency: Do the exercises six days a week. Take one rest day.
Intensity: Do water warm-up. In addition to the exercises you did in week 4, add one or two exercises each week until you are doing all the movements shown in this chapter.
Duration: Do four sets of 10 repetitions for each exercise.

10
Elbows and Wrists

The elbow is actually two joints in one. The first is a
hinge that allows you to bend and straighten your arm,
just like the knee allows you to bend and straighten
your leg. The other joint is designed to let you rotate
your lower arm and permits you to turn your wrist almost 180 degrees.

The hinge joint occurs where the ulna and radius, the
bones of the forearm, meet the humerus, the bone of
the upper arm. This joint has an interesting snag in its
construction. A little knob on the humerus, the trochlear, acts as a cam to angle the forearm slightly outward as it is extended. To see what we mean, extend
your arm with your palm turned upward. Notice that
the forearm curves slightly away from the body (toward the thumb). The position of the trochlear causes
this curve, which in everyday life may actually help you
when carrying a heavy bucket (in fact, this curve is
called the "carrying angle"). Throwing, however, really
brings out the weakness in this curved design by putting exceptional stress on the side of the joint where the

humerus and ulna meet. Baseball players, especially pitchers, and javelin throwers are plagued by tears and strains in the tendons that link muscle to bone in this area.

The second joint in the elbow is called the radioulnar joint, which, as you may have guessed, is the point where the radius and ulna meet. The ulna is a large, stationary bone. The radius, the smaller of the two forearm bones, pivots on the ulna, allowing you to pronate your forearm (turn it inward) and supinate it (turn it outward). When this joint is turned in conjunction with the shoulder joint, you can turn your wrist and hand almost a full 360 degrees.

Two of the elbow's most prominent features are pain centers when it comes to common elbow injuries. If you extend your arm with the palm up, the bump on the inside of your arm is your medial epicondyle and the one on the outside is your lateral epicondyle. The muscles of your forearm are attached by their tendons to these bony structures. (These are the muscles that let you flex and bend your wrist to move your hand up and down.) The most common elbow injuries will cause pain at these points.

The main muscles of the upper arm, the brachialis, triceps, and biceps (which is the one that forms that big bump when you flex your arm like Charles Atlas), attach at the elbow. These are the muscles that allow you to bend and straighten your elbow. The numerous muscles of the forearm attach at the wrist and elbow. These are the muscles that allow you to turn your wrist, as well as turn your forearm, in so many directions. When these muscles are weak, the force of your effort is transferred to the tendons that attach these muscles to bone. Like so many injuries, strengthening the muscles—in this case, the muscles of the upper and lower arm—is your best defense against reinjury. If your muscles are strong, the tendons are much less likely to become irritated, inflamed, or—worse yet—torn.

THE WRIST

The wrist is the smallest and most intricate joint in our body. No less than ten bones work together to give this joint its remarkable range of motion. The radius and ulna are two of these bones. They are linked by a complex system of ligaments and tendons to eight small bones, called the carpal bones, that are lined up in the wrist in two rows. The carpal bones slide in relation to one another, giving the wrist its flexibility independent of the forearm. The radius, as we have just described, turns the hand with its pivoting motion.

Most of the wrist muscles originate in the forearm. They begin at the elbow joint, cross the wrist, and are joined to the hand by tendons. These muscles are responsible for turning and bending the wrist, and they allow us to grip. While all this movement is important, these muscles also provide another important function. They stabilize the wrist, keeping it in place when we do fine motor movements such as writing, tying our shoes, or threading a needle. Imagine trying to do any of these activities with your wrist flopping around.

WATER EXERCISE FOR ELBOW AND WRIST INJURIES

An injury to the wrist or elbow causes a weakening of these forearm muscles. The exercises that follow are specifically designed to strengthen these muscles. There are also exercises to strengthen the upper arm muscles that are responsible for flexing and extending the elbow joint. The entire arm tends to be weakened by wrist and elbow injuries because the pain causes you to limit movement in both joints, so even if your injury is in your wrist, you should include these elbow flexion and extension exercises.

ELBOW AND WRIST INJURIES

Elbow and wrist injuries have one thing in common: the pain they bring will force your arm muscles into inactivity. Since these injuries may indicate that your arm muscles were not as strong as they should have been for your sport, inactivity is going to exacerbate this problem. Once your pain has subsided, you'll want to get in the pool and start your rebuilding program. The exercises in this chapter are designed to help you recover from the following injuries.

Tennis Elbow (Lateral Epicondylitis)

This injury is the bane of amateur tennis players. We say amateur because most professional players have sufficient forearm strength to use proper tennis technique. Tennis elbow is an inflammation of the tendons that join the forearm muscles to the lateral epicondyle (the bump on the outside of your elbow). This inflammation usually occurs because of improper use of the forearm muscles during the backhand stroke. As the player hits the ball, the wrist twists, putting excessive stress on these muscles. This stress is passed on to the weakest link, the tendons that join the muscles to the bone. The first thing most physicians will tell you is to take a break from tennis and give the tendons a chance to heal. These forearm-strengthening exercises will help you rehabilitate an injury while you are away from the tennis court. Strong forearm muscles will help stabilize your wrist joint and reduce your risk of a repeat bout with this insidious injury.

Medial Epicondylitis

This is like tennis elbow, only it's on the other side of the joint. Tendons that link forearm muscles to the medial

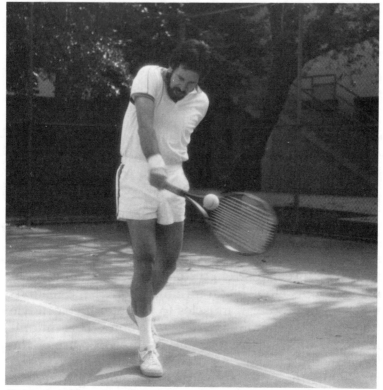

Proper backhand technique and strong forearm muscles will pre-vent tennis elbow.

epicondyle become inflamed or torn, usually because of overuse. This injury is common in sports that involve throwing, especially among baseball pitchers. Strong forearm muscles, in particular those that flex the wrist, will reduce the risk of a recurrence of the injury.

Radial Head Fracture

The most common cause of this injury is a fall on an outstretched hand. The force of the fall is transferred to the head of the radius in the elbow joint. This is a serious injury, and it should be treated by a physician. The radius is responsible for the twisting of the hand, and if the bone does not heal in the correct position, these movements may be limited. Recovery from this fracture may mean several weeks with your arm in a sling. After the bone has healed, these arm-strengthening exercises will be a welcome first step toward rehabilitating your weakened muscles.

Elbow Dislocation

This injury is usually caused by a blow to the arm that forces the elbow to hyperextend—that is, the elbow is straightened far past a healthy point. It is more common in contact sports such as football, rugby, and wrestling. The radius and ulna are forced off the humerus and incredible pain and swelling result. Your arm will probably be immobilized for several weeks, which, of course, will cause the muscles to weaken. Strengthening those muscles will help ensure your return to full range of motion in the joint.

Navicular Fracture

The tiny navicular, also called the scaphoid, is one of the eight carpal bones in your wrist. It sits just below your thumb and can be fractured if you fall on an outstretched hand. Again, it is common in contact sports such as football, rugby, and wrestling. Gymnasts and ice skaters are also at risk if they fall during their routine. Once it has been diagnosed—and this can be a challenge because the fracture may not show up on an x-ray—your physician will put your wrist in a cast. After the bone has healed, you can begin your strengthening exercises.

Wrist Sprain

The repeated turning of the wrist in sports such as tennis, squash, badminton, raquetball, and rowing can inflame the tendons or ligaments in your wrist. These connective tissues can also be torn or stretched if you fall on an outstretched hand. Strengthening the muscles in the forearm that turn the wrist will help prevent reinjury.

THE EXERCISES

Never do exercises that cause pain in the joint, especially at the site of your injury. Follow the workout guidelines presented in chapter 4.

Warm-Up
Water Cycling or Water Jogging, as described on pages 35 and 36.

I. Double-Arm Pulls
Body parts strengthened: front of upper arm (biceps, brachialis).

Stand in shoulder-deep water with legs apart at shoulder width and knees slightly bent. Begin with arms straight down at your sides. With palms facing upward, raise both hands toward your body, bringing them as close to your upper body as you can without discomfort. Keep elbows and upper arms next to your sides. Relax and slowly lower forearms to the starting position. This completes one repetition.

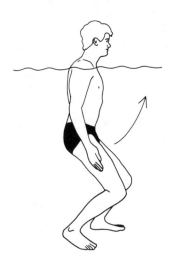

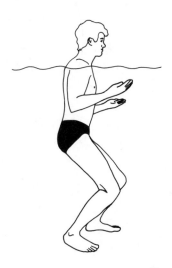

2. Wrist Figure Eights

Body parts strengthened: forearm (flexor carpi radialis, flexor carpi ulnaris, palmaris longus, extensor carpi ulnaris, extensor carpi radialis longus and brevis, extensor digitorum).

Stand in chest-deep water with your legs apart at shoulder width and knees slightly bent. Bend your right elbow 90 degrees. Keep the elbow tucked into your side. Begin with your right palm facing toward the pool bottom. Using the tip of your middle finger as a "pen," draw a sideways figure eight with your hand, moving only the wrist joint. One figure eight equals one repetition. Complete ten repetitions and then repeat with the left wrist. This equals one set.

Note: Keep your elbow and forearm in place. Don't move your hand with your forearm. The movement is all in the wrist.

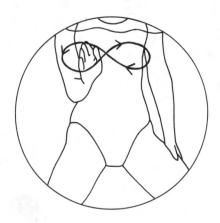

3. Double-Arm Pushes
Body parts strengthened:
back of upper arm (triceps).

Stand in chest-deep water with legs apart at shoulder width and knees slightly bent. Bend elbows to 90 degrees and turn palms toward the bottom of the pool. Keeping elbows and arms close to the sides of the body, push your hands down until they are at your sides. Relax and slowly raise forearms to the 90-degree starting position. This completes one repetition.

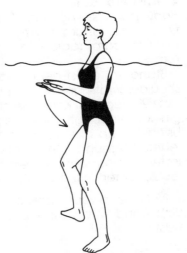

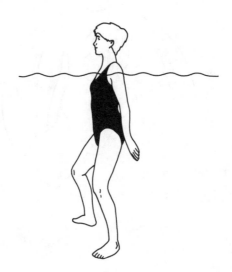

4. Wrist Alphabet

Body parts strengthened: forearm (flexor carpi radialis, flexor carpi ulnaris, palmaris longus, extensor carpi ulnaris, extensor carpi radialis longus and brevis, extensor digitorum).

Stand in chest-deep water with your legs apart at shoulder width and knees slightly bent. Bend your right elbow 90 degrees. Keep the elbow tucked into your side. Begin with your right palm facing toward the pool bottom. Using the tip of your middle finger as a "pen," draw the letters A through J, the first ten letters of the alphabet. Each letter is one repetition. Ten letters with the right hand followed by ten with the left equals one set.

Note: Keep your elbow and forearm in place. Don't move your hand with your forearm. The movement is all in the wrist.

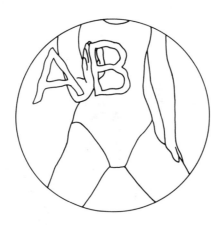

5. Forearm Sweeps

Body parts strengthened: front of upper arm (biceps, brachialis); back of upper arm (triceps).

Stand in neck-deep water with your legs apart at shoulder width and slightly bent. Extend your arms out to the sides at shoulder height and parallel to the bottom of the pool. Turn your palms forward. Bend your arms, bringing your forearm and hands to your chest. Keeping your elbows up and pushing against the water with the backs of your hands, return to the starting position. Push against the water with equal vigor as you move the hands toward and away from the chest. The completion of one inward and then outward sweep of the forearms equals one repetition.

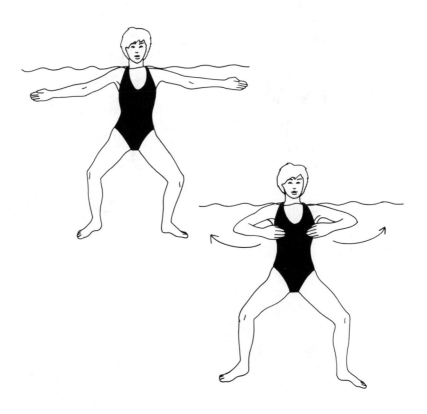

6. Hand Lifts

Body parts strengthened: forearm (flexor carpi radialis, flexor carpi ulnaris, palmaris longus).

Wearing swimmer's paddles on the palm side of each hand, stand in chest-deep water with legs apart at shoulder width and knees slightly bent. Bend elbows to 90 degrees and tuck them into your sides with the palms of your hands facing the surface. Lift your hands upward as far as possible using the wrist joint only. Relax and lower hands to the starting position. Each lift equals one repetition.

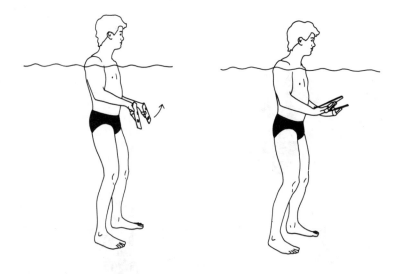

7. Reverse Hand Lifts

Body parts strengthened: forearm (extensor carpi ulnaris, extensor carpi radialis longus and brevis).

Wearing swimmer's paddles on the back of each hand, stand in chest-deep water with legs apart at shoulder width and knees slightly bent. Bend elbows to 90 degrees and tuck them into your sides with the backs of your hands toward the surface. Lift your hands upward as far as possible using the wrist joint only. Relax and lower hands to the starting position. Each lift equals one repetition.

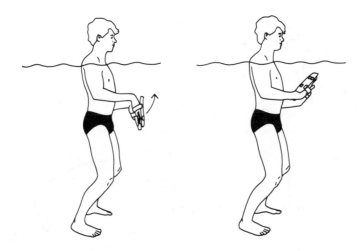

8. Pancake Flips

Body parts strengthened: forearm (extensor carpi radialis longus and brevis, flexor carpi radialis).

You will need a kitchen utensil, a plastic or metal flipper, for this exercise. Stand in chest-deep water with your legs apart at shoulder width and knees slightly bent. Hold the flipper in your right hand with your thumb up, as if you were going to flip a pancake. Bend your right elbow to 90 degrees and tuck it into your side. Raise your hand—and the flipper—bending only the wrist. Relax and lower your hand to starting position. Each time you lift the flipper you have done one repetition. Complete ten repetitions and then repeat with the left wrist. This equals one set.

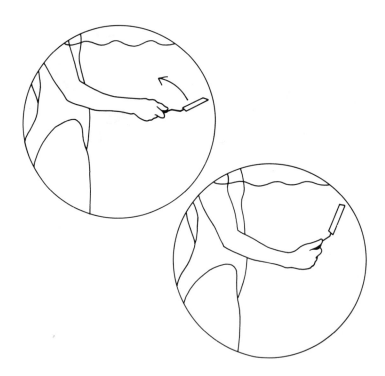

9. Backhand Pancake Flips

Body parts strengthened: forearm (extensor carpi ulnaris, flexor carpi ulnaris).

Use a metal or plastic pancake flipper for this exercise. Stand in chest-deep water with your legs apart at shoulder width and knees slightly bent. With your right arm straight down at your side, hold the flipper so that it points behind you with the broad side facing the surface. The back of your hand is facing away from your body. Bend your wrist, lifting your hand and the flipper upward. Relax and return to the starting position. This is one repetition. Complete ten repetitions and then repeat with the left wrist. This equals one set.

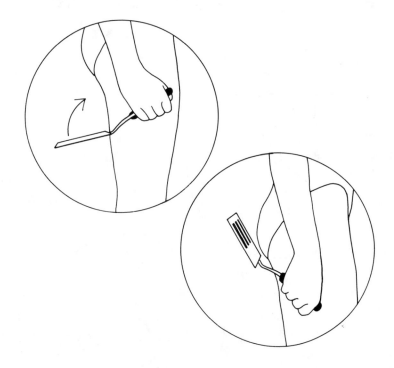

10. Inward Wrist Turns

Body parts strengthened: forearm (pronator quadratus, pronator teres).

Stand in chest-deep water with your legs apart at shoulder width and knees slightly bent. Bend your right elbow to 90 degrees and tuck it into your side. Hold the flipper vertically in your right hand with the flipping side facing toward the midline of your body. Rotate your wrist and hand inward as far as possible. At the bottom of the turn, the flipping side of the flipper should be facing the pool bottom. Rotate back to the starting position to complete one repetition. After ten repetitions, repeat with the left arm. This equals one set.

Note: Turn the flipper with your wrist and forearm only. Don't use your upper arm or shoulder. Keep your elbow bent and tucked into your side.

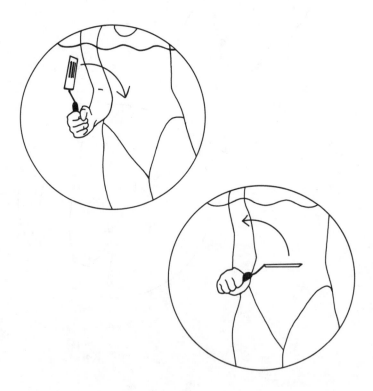

11. Outward Wrist Turns

Body parts strengthened: forearm (supinator).

Stand in chest-deep water. Bend your elbow to 90 de-grees and tuck it into your side. Hold the flipper vertically in your right hand with the flipping side facing away from your body. Rotate your wrist and hand outward as far as possi-ble. At the bottom of the turn, the flipping side of the flipper should be toward the pool bottom. Rotate back to the start-ing position to complete one repetition. After ten repeti-tions, repeat with the left arm. This equals one set.

Note: Turn the flipper with your wrist and forearm only. Don't use your upper arm or shoulder. Keep your elbow bent and tucked into your side.

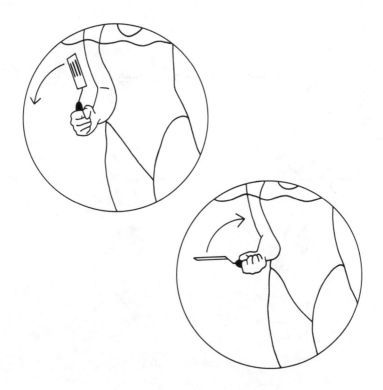

ELBOW AND WRIST WORKOUT

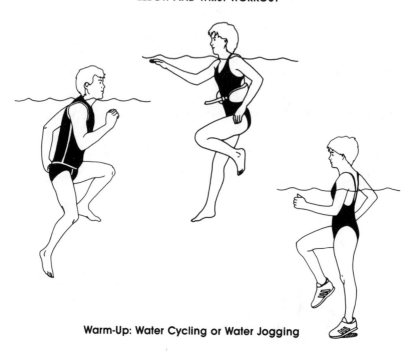

Warm-Up: Water Cycling or Water Jogging

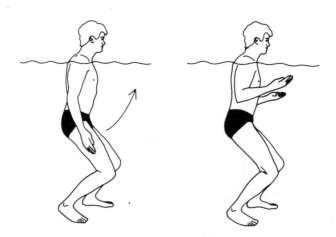

I. Double-Arm Pulls

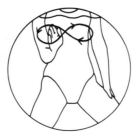

2. Wrist Figure Eights

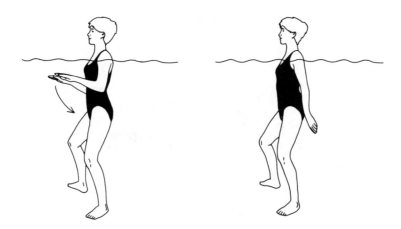

3. Double-Arm Pushes

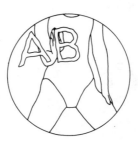

4. Wrist Alphabet

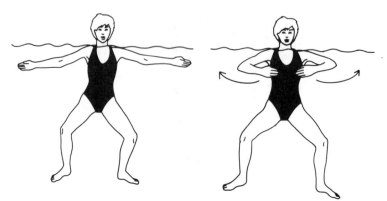

5. Forearm Sweeps

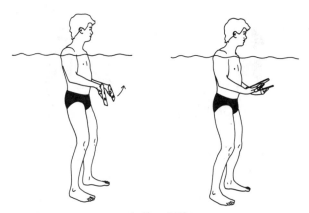

6. Hand Lifts

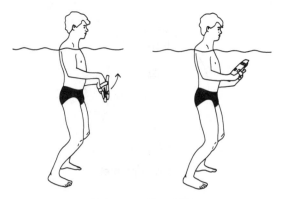

7. Reverse Hand Lifts

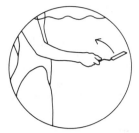
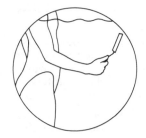

8. Pancake Flips

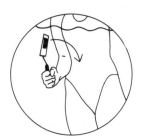
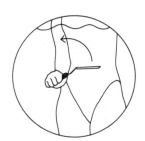

9. Backhand Pancake Flips

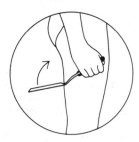
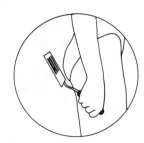

10. Inward Wrist Turns

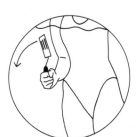
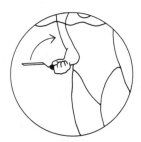

11. Outward Wrist Turns

WORKOUT SCHEDULE

Weeks 1 and 2
Frequency: Do the exercises three days a week with at least one rest day between training sessions.
Intensity: Do water warm-up and the first three exercises in this chapter.
Duration: Do two sets of 10 repetitions for each exercise.

Weeks 3 and 4
Frequency: Do the exercises five days a week with two rest days. Don't take two rest days in a row.
Intensity: Do water warm-up. In addition to the three exercises you did in weeks 1 and 2, add two exercises per week to the program.
Duration: Do three sets of 10 repetitions for each exercise.

Weeks 5 to 8
Frequency: Do the exercises six days a week. Take one rest day.
Intensity: Do water warm-up. In addition to the exercises you did in week 4, add one or two exercises each week until you are doing all the movements shown in this chapter.
Duration: Do four sets of 10 repetitions for each exercise.

11
The Total-Body Water Workout

Once you are healthy and participating in sports, you do not have to give up pool exercise. The pool can continue to be an effective training location, especially for the aerobic conditioning phase of your workouts. Running, one of the most common forms of aerobic training, is a high-impact activity—if it is done on dry land. When you run, your foot strikes the ground with an impact of three to five times your weight: the equivalent of approximately 700 pounds of pressure for a 150-pound man. The constant pounding of the body while running causes injury to your joints and soft tissues—so much so that it is almost impossible to avoid injury if you run high weekly mileage over many years. Your feet, ankles, knees, and back just can't take that kind of abuse.

The pool-running program shown here won't replace running on land. Let's face it, the scenery doesn't change much when you run in the deep end of the pool. But if, like many other athletes who run regularly, you

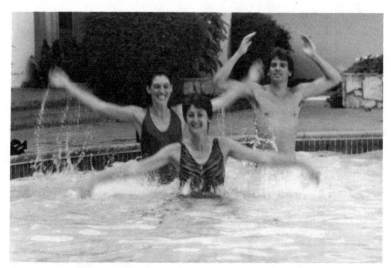

Aerobic water exercise improves the efficiency of your heart, lungs, and circulatory system.

replace some of your weekly mileage with a workout in the pool, you'll reduce the stress on your body, cut down your risk of injury, and still enjoy all the fitness benefits of running for aerobic conditioning.

WHAT IS AEROBIC CONDITIONING?

Aerobic exercise makes your heart, lungs, and circulatory system more efficient. Research has shown that it reduces risk of coronary heart disease and stroke and that it lowers blood pressure and helps create healthy levels of blood cholesterol. Besides these important physiological benefits, studies have shown that individuals who do regular aerobic exercise feel better, sleep better, have improved self-image, suffer less from anxiety and depression, and can cope with stress more effectively. This is the kind of exercise that is important to your physical and mental health. Everyone from young athletes to senior citizens can enjoy the benefits of aerobic exercise.

To attain the fitness and health benefits of aerobic exercise you must work out within what experts refer to as your *training heart rate range.* When your heart is beating at a certain rate—and this rate varies from person to person—it is working at an aerobic level that will improve your fitness. The American College of Sports Medicine research shows that if you exercise within your training heart rate range three to five times a week for a minimum of fifteen minutes, you will experience the mental and physical benefits of aerobic exercise.

CALCULATING YOUR TRAINING RANGE

Determining your heart rate range for aerobic training takes a few minutes of simple calculations. First, you need to find out your resting pulse. Take your pulse for one minute in the morning, before you get out of bed. You do this by placing your index and middle finger on your radial artery, which is close to your thumb on the

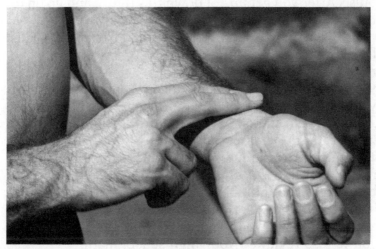

Take your pulse on your radial artery by placing your fingertips on your wrist as shown.

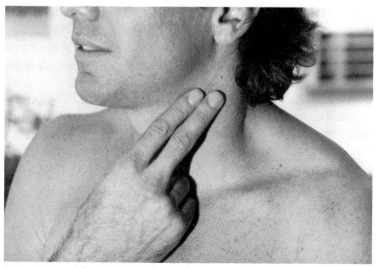

Place your fingertips on your neck, as shown, to take your pulse on your carotid artery.

inside of your wrist, or on your carotid artery, just under your chin. The photograph here and on page 177 shows the proper position for taking your pulse. Your morning pulse is your minimum heart rate, or resting pulse. After you get up, jot down this figure and go on to the rest of the calculation.

Your next step is to subtract your age from 220. This figure is your maximum heart rate. Now subtract the minimum from the maximum heart rate. This figure is your heart rate reserve. Calculate 60 and 90 percent of your heart rate reserve by multiplying this number by .6 and .9. Add the 60-percent figure to your minimum heart rate (the resting pulse you took in the morning). This number is the *low end* of your training heart rate range. Now add the 90-percent figure to your minimum heart rate. That number is the *top end* of your training heart rate range. Not only do you now know the high and low end of your training heart rate range, but you've also reviewed your high school math.

The following chart gives you the steps in order as well as a sample calculation.

   220
-   minus your age
- =   equals maximum heart rate
- −   minus your resting heart rate
- =   equals maximum heart rate reserve
- ×   times .6
- =   equals 60 percent of your maximum heart rate reserve
- +   plus your resting pulse
- =   equals the *low end* of your training heart rate range

   220
- −   minus your age
- =   equals maximum heart rate
- −   minus your resting heart rate
- =   equals maximum heart rate reserve
- ×   times .9
- =   equals 90 percent of your maximum heart rate reserve
- +   plus your resting pulse
- =   equals the *high end* of your training heart rate range

Calculation for a 35-year-old with a resting pulse of 65 beats per minute:

   220
- −   35   minus your age
- =   185   equals maximum heart rate
- −   65   minus your resting heart rate
- =   120   equals maximum heart rate reserve
- ×   .6   times .6
- =   72   equals 60 percent of your maximum heart rate reserve
- +   65   plus your resting pulse
- =   137   equals the *low end* of your training heart rate range

	220	
−	35	minus your age
=	185	equals maximum heart rate
−	65	minus your resting heart rate
=	120	equals maximum heart rate reserve
×	.9	times .9
=	108	equals 90 percent of your maximum heart rate reserve
+	65	plus your resting pulse
=	173	equals the *high end* of your training heart rate range

You now know your personal training heart rate range for aerobic exercise. When you are doing the aerobic pool workouts, take your pulse midway through your workout and immediately after finishing the workout. You do this by placing your fingertips on the carotid or radial arteries and counting your heartbeats for ten seconds. Multiply this number by six and you know your heartbeat for sixty seconds.

When you are doing your aerobic training, your heart rate should be within the training range. If you regularly monitor your pulse during your aerobic exercise on land, you will find your heart rate is slightly lower in the pool even though you feel as though you are exerting the same effort. Recent research has shown that the heart rate will be eight to ten beats per minute lower in the water than it would be at the same level of exertion on land. This occurs because of the physiological effects of buoyancy and water pressure on the circulatory system and heart. As long as you are within your training heart rate range, you will enjoy the benefits of aerobic exercise.

AEROBIC POOL WORKOUTS

We have included two types of workouts in this program. The first is a highly enjoyable *contact* workout, which means that as you do it, your feet touch the bottom of the pool. This program may take you back to the days when you used to splash and bob around the pool as a child. Unlike the running workouts, which, as their name implies, involve only the running motion, the contact workout has a variety of exercises. It is designed to strengthen and tone the major muscle groups of the body and improve your aerobic fitness.

The running workouts are *noncontact*, meaning you do them in the deep end of the pool. Pool running allows you to maintain your aerobic conditioning while you are still injured. You are not in contact with the pool bottom, so there is no impact stress on your muscles and joints. As long as pool running does not cause pain at the site of your injury, you can use this method of conditioning to maintain your aerobic fitness during your recovery.

When your injury has healed, you can use the pool running or the contact aerobic program as a refreshing alternative to dryland aerobic activity, such as running, cycling, or aerobic dance.

CONTACT AEROBIC WORKOUT

Equipment

The following equipment will help you derive full benefit from the program:

1. A water-resistant watch, or a timer or clock, with a second hand (or display). You'll be able to time each of the exercises and take your pulse midway through and immediately after the workout.
2. Athletic shoes (optional). You may find your footing

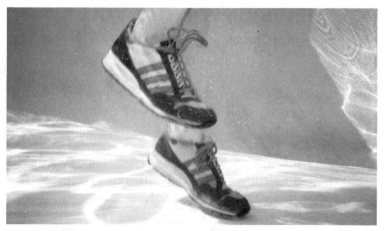

Wearing athletic shoes in the pool will give you more secure footing.

on the pool bottom is more secure if you wear athletic shoes.

3. Music. Your workout will be greatly enhanced if you have lively music playing as you exercise. Take your battery-operated tape player or radio to the pool with you. (Warning: avoid electrical shock. Do not use plug-in electrical equipment near water.)

CONTACT AEROBIC WORKOUT SCHEDULE

The nine exercises take fifteen minutes to complete, not including the warm-up and cool-down. This is the minimum length of time you must exercise to train aerobically, providing you are within your training heart rate range. To lengthen the workout, repeat the sequence of nine exercises to create a workout of thirty, forty-five, sixty minutes or more.

Frequency: Do this workout three to five times a week or in conjunction with your regular aerobic training. For example, you may want to run or cycle two days a week and do this contact aerobic pool workout on the third day.

Duration: A minimum of 15 minutes.

Intensity: Check your pulse midway through and immediately after the workout. Your heart rate should be within your training heart rate range.

Contact Aerobic Exercises

This exercise program has been designed to include all of the major muscles of the body. If you do this entire workout, you will not only develop aerobic fitness but strengthen and firm your muscles as well. These exercises involve the following body parts and muscles: calf (tibialis posterior, gastrocnemius, soleus); front of calf (tibialis anterior, extensor digitorum brevis, extensor hallucis longus); front of thigh (quadriceps); back of thigh (hamstrings); inner thigh (adductor longus, brevis, and magnus; pectineus; gracilis); hip (iliopsoas, sartorius, tensor fascia lata); buttocks (gluteus maximus, medius, and minimus); abdomen (rectus abdominis, internal and external obliques); back (erector spinae, trapezius, rhomboids); shoulder (latissimus dorsi, teres minor and major, deltoid, infraspinatus, supraspinatus, subscapularis); arm (biceps, triceps).

Warm-Up
Stand in chest-deep water. Run slowly from one side of the pool to the other.
Duration: continue for four to five minutes.

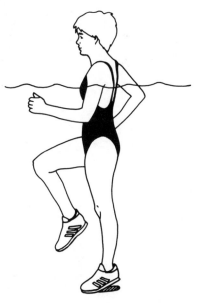

1. Sprinting in Place

Stand in chest-deep water. Run vigorously in place, bringing your knees up to the point at which your thighs are parallel with the pool bottom. Keep your arms bent at 90 degrees and bring your elbows back as you raise the opposite leg.

Duration: continue for two minutes.

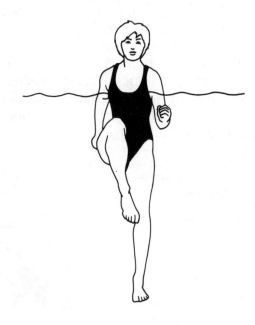

2. Jumping Jacks

Stand in chest-deep water with legs apart at shoulder width and knees slightly bent. Raise your arms over your head and keep them out of the water throughout the exercise. Jump up and, as you do, bring your legs together. Immediately spread them apart again, landing with your legs apart at shoulder width and knees slightly bent. *Don't touch the bottom of the pool when your legs are together. Land with your legs apart.* Continue jumping, moving your legs inward and then outward.

Duration: continue for one minute.

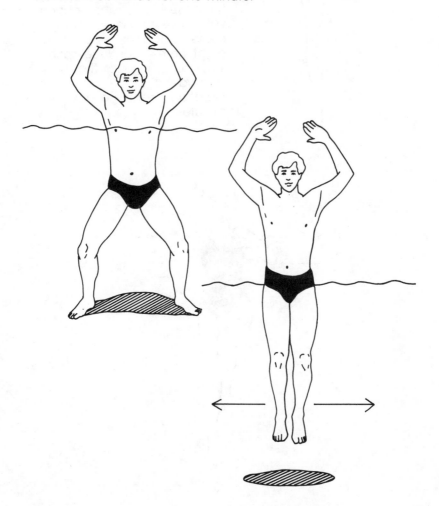

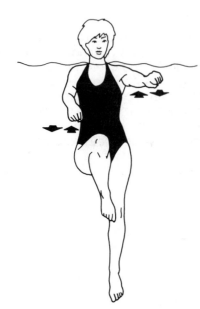

3. Run and Punch
Stand in shoulder-deep water. Sprint in place, punching your arms to the front, underwater, to a count of eight. As you raise your right knee, you punch the left arm forward. As you raise the left knee, you punch the right arm forward. Punch to the front eight times with each hand. Then continue sprinting and punch your arms to the side in the same manner, punching eight times. Continue sprinting, punching to the front and side.
Duration: continue for two minutes.

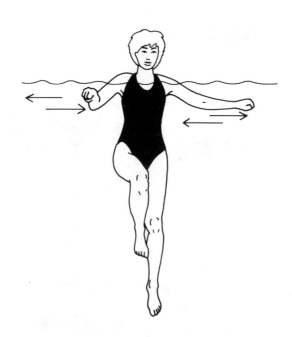

4. Lunges and Leaps

Stand in chest-deep water with your left knee bent and your weight over your left foot. The right leg is extended behind you. Jump up and, as you do, bring your right leg forward and extend the left leg behind you. Keep your arms bent at 90 degrees and move them as if you are sprinting, with the left arm back when the right leg is forward, right arm forward when the left leg is back.
Duration: continue for one minute.

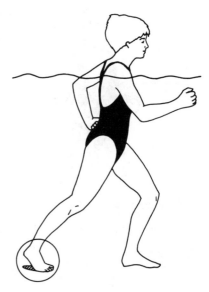

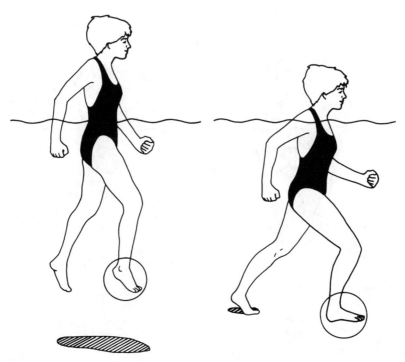

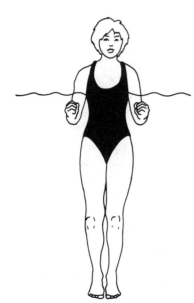

5. Front and Side Knee Lifts

Stand with legs together in chest-deep water. Raise your left knee four times, keeping the other leg straight. Rotate your leg to the side and raise your knee four times. Return to the starting position with both legs together. Raise the right knee four times to the front and then four times to the side. Continue raising one knee to the front and side, and then the other.

Duration: continue for two minutes.

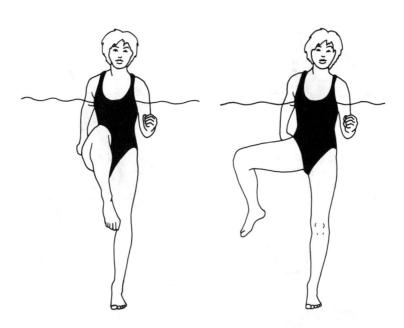

6. Bounding

Stand in chest-deep water with your back to the pool wall. Bound from one side of the pool to the other, driving your right knee forward as you push off with the left leg and foot. Then drive the left knee forward as you push off with the right leg and foot. Keep your arms bent at 90 degrees and move them vigorously forward and back, bringing the right arm forward as you drive the left knee forward, and the left arm forward with the right knee.
Duration: continue for two minutes.

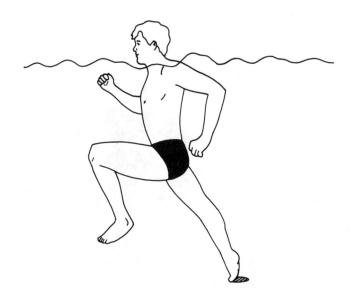

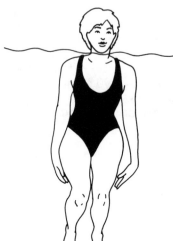

7. Double-Leg Jumps
Stand in chest-deep water with legs together and knees slightly bent. Keep your arms at your sides. Jump up as high as you can. Bend your knees as you land and immediately do another jump.
Duration: continue for one minute.

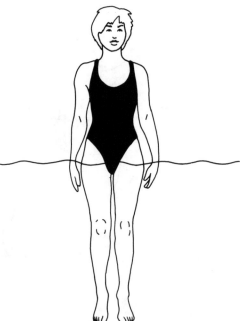

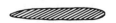

8. Squats and Arm Pulls

Stand in chest-deep water with legs straight and apart at shoulder width. Extend your arms out to the sides, your hands cupped and your palms turned downward. Bend your legs into a squat position and, as you do, bring your arms down and in front of your torso. Straighten your legs, raising your arms as you do. Repeat this movement three times to the front. Then bring your arms behind your torso as you squat, raising them to the the surface as you straighten your legs. Continue bending and straightening your legs, three times with your arms moving to the front and three times to the back.

Duration: continue for two minutes.

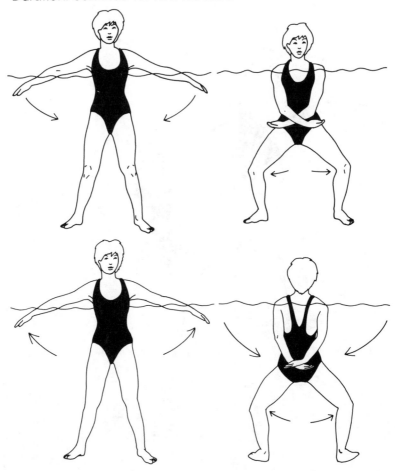

9. Twisting

Stand in chest-deep water with body erect. Bend your arms 90 degrees, and face both palms in the same direction so one thumb points up and one thumb points down. Jump up and turn your legs and body to the right. As you do, sweep your arms in the opposite direction, pushing against the water with your hands. After you land, jump up and twist to the left. Turn your hands and arms, sweeping your hands to the right as you twist.

Duration: continue for two minutes.

Take your pulse. Is it within your training heart rate range?

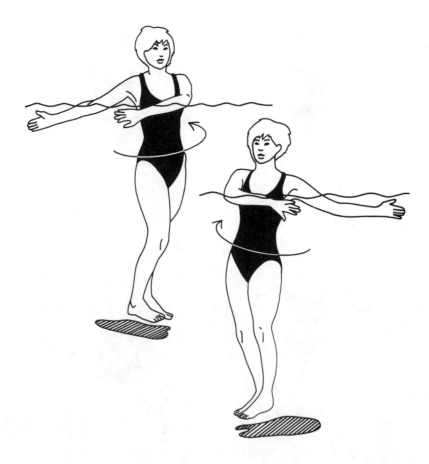

Cool-Down
Jog slowly from one side of
the pool to the other for five
minutes, then proceed to the
total-body stretching program outlined in the next
chapter.

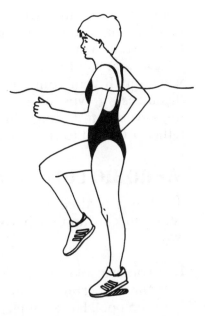

NONCONTACT WORKOUT:
WATER RUNNING

If you are injured, the running you do on dry land will
be eliminated or reduced during your recovery time.
You must replace these missed workouts with pool running. Whether you are a football player who includes
forty-yard uphill sprints in his daily workout—or a tri-
athlete who runs hundreds of road miles a week—your
running program can be duplicated in the pool.

A program of water running is also an excellent starting point for the beginner. If you are overweight or taking up exercise after a long period of inactivity, water
running is a safe and effective way to get started.

What Is Water Running?

Water running workouts take place in the deep end of
the pool. Wearing a flotation device to keep your head

above the water line, you run, just as if you were on dry land. If long-distance running is your usual program or if you want to maintain or improve your cardiovascular fitness, you run for fifteen minutes or more after your warm-up. If your running program involves short, fast distances—a type of running called "interval training"—you can do these in the pool with the help of a tether attached to the side of the pool.

AEROBIC LONG-DISTANCE WORKOUT

If running is already part of your weekly workout on land you can approach your pool workouts in three ways:

1. If you are not injured and you want to stay that way, replace a certain amount of your mileage with time in the pool. For example, if you run for half an hour four days a week, spend one of those days running for half an hour in the pool.
2. If your workouts include a variety of aerobic activities—such as cycling, running, and aerobic dance—replace one of these dry-land workouts with water running once a week. You'll maintain cardiovascular fitness and reduce your risk of injury by greatly reducing the stress on your joints and muscles.
3. If you are injured, do all of your running in the pool until your injury is better. When you have recovered, continue to do some aerobic training in the deep end of the pool if you want to stay healthy.

You will maintain and improve your cardiovascular fitness with water running, provided you train within your training heart rate range. Check your pulse while you are running in the deep end and right after finishing your workout to be sure you are working at this level. If you are below the low end of your training heart rate range, run faster. If you are above the high end of your range, slow down.

Equipment

You'll need a pool with a deep end. In addition, your equipment should include:

1. A flotation device, preferably one that leaves your arms and legs free to do a natural running motion. A waterskiing belt, waterskiing vest, or the Wet Vest®, a product designed specifically for water running workouts, are all excellent.
2. A water-resistant watch, or a timer or clock, with a second hand (or display) so you can time your work-out and take your pulse. There are a wide variety of

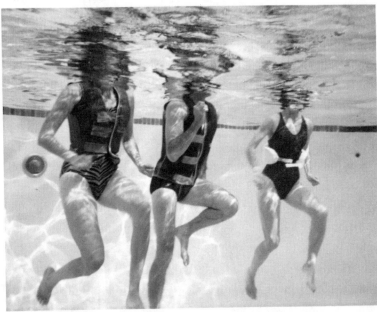

A group of long-distance runners gets together to do some of their weekly mileage in the pool.

water-resistant sports watches available today. You can buy a twenty-five-dollar digital watch that will time your workout and "beep" you when it's over.

3. Music. Water running can be tedious, so how about some entertainment? Take your battery-operated tape player or radio to the pool with you.

4. Training partner. Whether you are on land or in the pool, it's a lot easier to stick with your program and a lot more fun if you run with a friend.

Technique

When you run in the water, your body position should be the same as on land. Run with your body upright in the water. When you are learning, there is a tendency to bend at the waist. Keep your torso over your legs and your head over your neck. Move your arms back and forth, bringing the elbows well back. Lift your knees until your thighs are nearly parallel to the pool bottom.

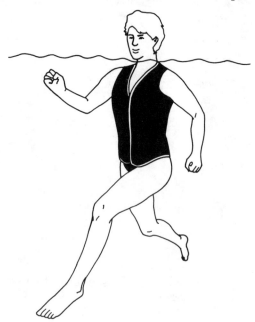

AEROBIC LONG-DISTANCE
WORKOUT SCHEDULE

If you are overweight, injury prone, or a beginning exerciser, the following six-week aerobic water running workout is an excellent exercise program for improving your aerobic condition.

Weeks 1 and 2

Warm-Up: Jog slowly for four minutes in the deep end.
Frequency: Do this workout three days a week with at least one rest day between aerobic running workouts.
Duration: Run for 15 minutes.
Intensity: Check your pulse during the workout to be sure you are working within your training heart rate range. If your pulse is too low, run more quickly; if it is too high, reduce speed.

Weeks 3 and 4

Warm-up: Jog slowly for four minutes in the deep end.
Frequency: Four days a week with three rest days. Do not do four days training in a row.
Duration: Run for 20 minutes during week 3; 30 minutes during week 4.
Intensity: Check your pulse during the workout to be sure you are working within your training heart rate range. If your pulse is too low, run more quickly; if it is too high, reduce speed.

Weeks 5 and 6

Warm-Up: Jog slowly for four minutes in the deep end.
Frequency: Five days a week with two rest days.
Duration: Run 40 minutes during week 5; 50 minutes during week 6.
Intensity: Check your pulse during the workout to be sure you are working within your training heart rate range. If your pulse is too low, run more quickly; if it is too high, reduce speed.

DEEP-END SPRINTING

If your sport involves sprint training, this too can be done in the deep end of the pool. When you are injured, sprinting in the pool will take the stress off your injury and allow you to maintain your sprinting form and fitness.

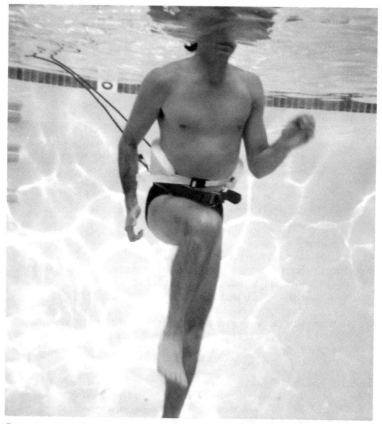

Deep-end sprinting on a tether lets you "run" at high speeds without putting stress on your bones, joints, and muscles.

Sprint training is not aerobic. It involves running at full tilt for a short time, resting for a few seconds, and then sprinting again. This type of conditioning is necessary for sports that involve short, explosive bursts of speed, such as volleyball, football, and baseball. The sprint/rest/sprint technique is called *interval training*, meaning you have a set interval of effort and rest.

The best way to sprint in the pool is to run against a tether. The best homemade tether is a twenty-five-foot piece of surgical tubing—the elastic, durable type of tubing used by physicians. Loop this through a cloth belt that is securely fastened around your waist, positioning the tether at the middle of your back. As you sprint, the other end of the tether is held by a training partner on the pool deck or tied to the pool ladder. You run against the resistance of the tubing, which allows you to move your arms and legs rapidly without bumping into the side of the pool.

Sprinting Technique

Float in the middle of the deep end. Wear a flotation device and position the belt and tether as shown. As you sprint, move your legs and arms vigorously, just as you would on dry land. You may angle your body slightly, as if leaning into the motion on land. Keep your knee lift high and move your arms vigorously back and forth,

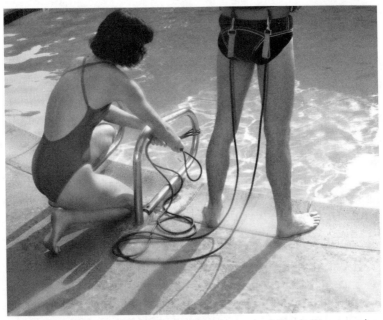

During the sprint-interval workout, one end of the tether can be tied to the ladder, or your training partner can hold the tether while standing on the pool deck.

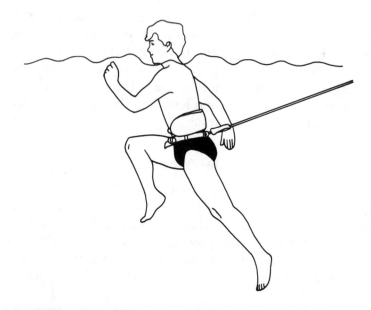

keeping the elbows bent at 90 degrees. Don't bend at the waist. Check your body position. Keep your torso in alignment with your legs.

Caution: Interval running in the pool is challenging and tiring. Never do these workouts without a training partner. There must be someone at the pool who can assist you if you become overly fatigued.

Interval Training Workouts

You can approach your pool interval-training program in three ways:

1. If you are injured, do your sprint training in the deep end of the pool until you have recovered. For example, if you usually run five 70-second, 400-meter sprints with 60 seconds rest between each sprint, duplicate these times in the pool.

2. Even if you are not injured, you can reduce the stress of your sprint workouts by doing some of your weekly interval work in the deep end.
3. If you want to add explosive, high-speed running to your long-distance water running workouts, do the interval workouts on the days you are not doing deep-end aerobic running. (Interval workouts are not aerobic because your heart rate drops during the rest period. For aerobic training to be effective, your heart rate must stay within your training heart rate range continuously for a minimum of fifteen minutes.)

INTERVAL TRAINING WORKOUT SCHEDULE

Do the interval sprint workout after you have completed one of the six-week aerobic water workout programs described earlier. Do these workouts on the days you are not doing your aerobic water running or after

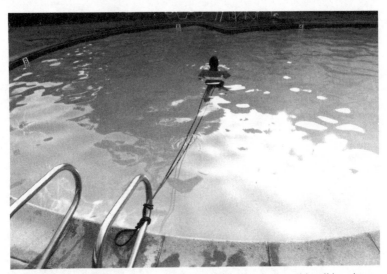

Rest between sprint intervals by floating, slowly "walking" in place, or treading water.

you have finished your aerobic running. These workouts can be done up to four times a week, provided you have a rest day between workouts.

Beginner: Weeks 1 and 2

Warm-Up: Jog slowly for four minutes in the deep end.

Duration: Do six 15-second sprints resting for 60 seconds between sprints. You may rest by "walking" slowly in the water, treading water, or floating in place.

Intermediate: Weeks 3 and 4

Warm-Up: Jog slowly for four minutes in the deep end.

Duration: Do ten 30-second sprints, resting for 60 seconds between sprints. You may rest by "walking" slowly in the water, treading water, or floating in place.

Advanced: Weeks 5 and 6

Warm-Up: Jog slowly for four minutes in the deep end.

Duration: Do ten 30-second sprints, resting for 30 seconds between sprints. You may rest by "walking" slowly in the water, treading water, or floating in place.

TOTAL-BODY WATER WORKOUT

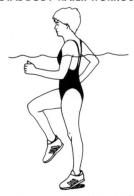

Warm-Up: Water Jogging—four to five minutes

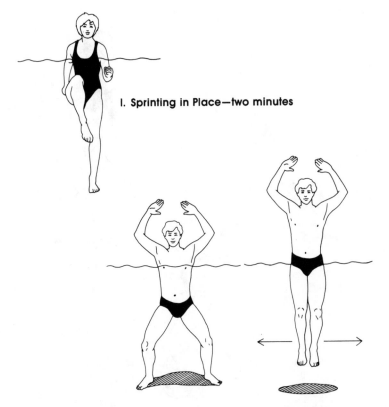

1. Sprinting in Place—two minutes

2. Jumping Jacks—one minute

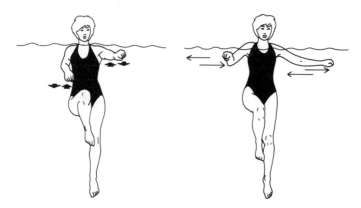

3. Run and Punch—two minutes

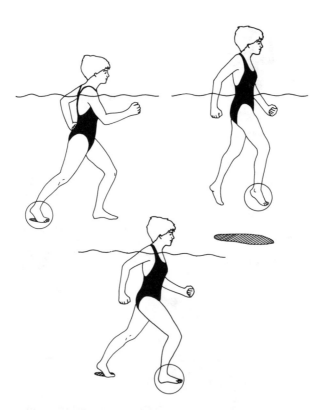

4. Lunges and Leaps—one minute

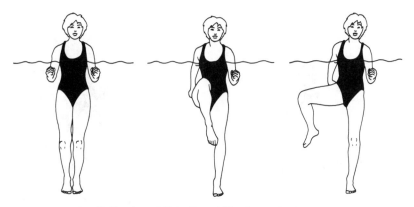

5. Front and Side Knee Lifts—two minutes

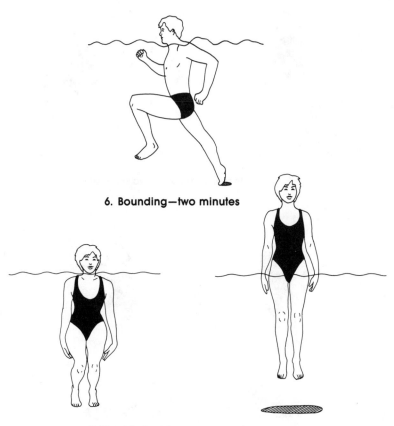

6. Bounding—two minutes

7. Double-Leg Jumps—one minute

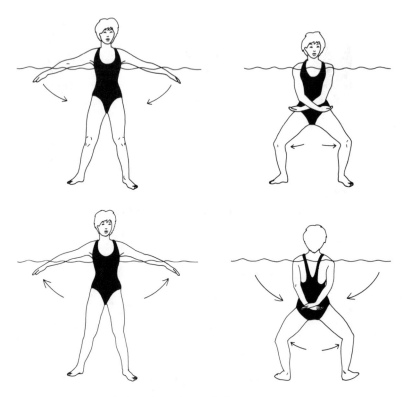

8. Squats and Arm Pulls—two minutes

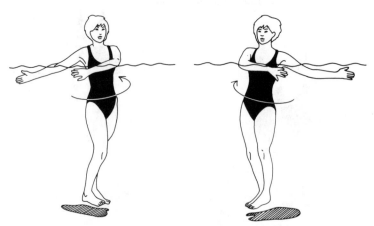

9. Twisting—two minutes

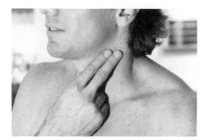

Take Your Pulse (photo)

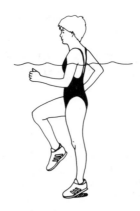

Cool-Down: Water Jogging—five minutes

CONTACT AEROBIC WORKOUT SCHEDULE

Frequency: Do this workout three to five times a week or in conjunction with your regular aerobic training.

Duration: A minimum of 15 minutes, not including the warm-up and cool-down. Time the aerobic movements only.

Intensity: Check your pulse. Your heart rate should be within your training heart rate range.

AEROBIC WATER RUNNING

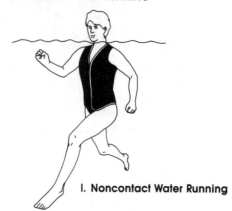

I. Noncontact Water Running

AEROBIC LONG-DISTANCE
WORKOUT SCHEDULE

Weeks 1 and 2
Warm-up: Jog slowly for 4 minutes in the deep end.
Frequency: Do this workout three days a week with at least one rest day between aerobic running workouts.
Duration: Run for 15 minutes.
Intensity: Check your pulse during the workout to be sure you are working within your training heart rate range. If your pulse is too low, run more quickly; if it is too high, reduce speed.

Weeks 3 and 4
Warm-up: Jog slowly for 4 minutes in the deep end.
Frequency: Four days a week with three rest days. Do not do four days training in a row.
Duration: Run for 20 minutes during week 3; 30 minutes during week 4.
Intensity: Check your pulse during the workout to be sure you are working within your training heart rate range. If your pulse is too low, run more quickly; if it is too high, reduce speed.

Weeks 5 and 6
Warm-Up: Jog slowly for four minutes in the deep end.
Frequency: Five days a week with two rest days.
Duration: Run 40 minutes during week 5, 50 minutes during week 6.
Intensity: Check your pulse during the workout to be sure you are working within your training heart rate range. If your pulse is too low, run more quickly; if it is too high, reduce speed.

DEEP-END SPRINTING WORKOUT

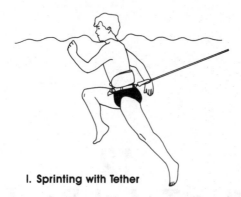

I. Sprinting with Tether

INTERVAL TRAINING WORKOUT SCHEDULE

Do the interval sprint workout after you have completed the six-week aerobic water workout program described earlier. Do these workouts on the days you are not doing your aerobic water running or after you have finished your aerobic running. These workouts can be done up to four times a week, provided you have a rest day between workouts.

Beginner: Weeks 1 and 2
Warm-Up: Jog slowly for four minutes in the deep end.
Duration: Do six 15-second sprints, resting for 60 seconds
                between sprints. You may rest by "walking" slowly
                in the water, treading water, or floating in place.

Intermediate: Weeks 3 and 4
Warm-Up: Jog slowly for four minutes in the deep end.
Duration: Do ten 30-second sprints, resting for 60 seconds
                between sprints. You may rest by "walking" slowly
                in the water, treading water, or floating in place.

Advanced: Weeks 5 and 6
Warm-Up: Jog slowly for four mintues in the deep end.
Duration: Do ten 30-second sprints, resting for 30 seconds
                between sprints. You may rest by "walking" slowly
                in the water, treading water, or floating in place.

12
The Total-Body Stretching Workout

Stretching in the pool is the perfect way to end your water workout, whether you are injured or doing one of the aerobic fitness programs described in the previous chapter. You will get the most out of any stretching program by doing it at the end of your workout, when the muscles are warm and the most pliable. Stretching will leave you in a calm and relaxed state of mind at the completion of your exercise session, as well as reduce the stiffness and soreness your workout may cause.

HOW TO STRETCH

Stretching is a noncompetitive, pain-free activity that is an important component of any well-balanced training program. This ten- to fifteen-minute stretching session will help you unwind after your workout, provided you use correct technique. Here are the steps to correct stretching:

1. Move slowly when you stretch. Don't bounce. The body has a reflex reaction to fast movements that

actually tightens, rather than loosens, your muscles. Moving slowly is the only way you can override this reflex and increase the elasticity of your muscles.

2. Stretch to the point of mild muscular tension, never pain. We all have different levels of flexibility, so don't compare your stretch to others. Trying to stretch to the point of pain will not increase your flexibility, and it may injure the muscles and joints.

3. Once you have stretched to the point of mild tension, hold that position for ten to thirty seconds. The longer you hold the stretch, the more you will increase the elasticity of the muscle tissue.

4. Breathe. As you hold the stretch, take in deep breaths and let them out slowly. Deep, controlled breathing increases muscular relaxation, which in turn allows the fibers to stretch more easily.

5. Stretching should be pleasant. If it causes pain, you're not doing it right. Enjoy your stretching. Follow the above steps and use the stretching movements to end your workout in a calm, relaxed state of mind.

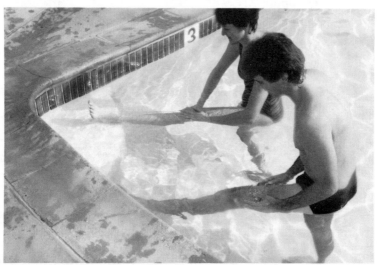

Stretching is a calm, relaxing way to end your pool workout.

Stretching in the water is a lot easier than on land because the water helps you balance. Therefore, these simple movements should cause you no pain or discomfort. If, however, you have an injury that is aggravated by any of these movements, do not include that movement in the program. Check with a sports physician or physical therapist before you try it again.

THE STRETCHES

WORKOUT SCHEDULE

Follow this schedule to get full benefit from your stretching program.

Frequency: Stretch at the conclusion of every pool workout.
Duration: Hold each stretch for 10 to 30 seconds.
Intensity: Move to the position at which you feel mild tension in your muscles, never pain. Hold that position for the duration of the stretch, breathing slowly and deeply and concentrating on relaxation.

1. Achilles Stretch

Body part stretched: calf (gastrocnemius, soleus).

Stand in the shallow end, facing the pool wall. Hold the wall with both hands. Extend your right leg straight behind you, keeping your heel on the floor of the pool. Bend your left knee, keeping your right knee straight, and lean into the wall with your entire body, bending your arms to increase the stretch in your calf if necessary. Hold the stretch. Relax. Repeat with leg positions reversed.

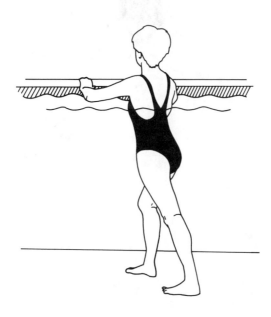

2. Inner Thigh Stretch

Body part stretched: inner thigh (adductor longus, brevis, and magnus; pectineus, gracilis).

Stand in the shallow end with your legs wide apart and arms extended out to the sides. Bend your left leg, placing the weight of your body over the left leg. Stretch your right leg out to the side, keeping the leg straight and the foot pointing forward. Hold the stretch. Relax. Repeat with your right leg bent, stretching the left leg.

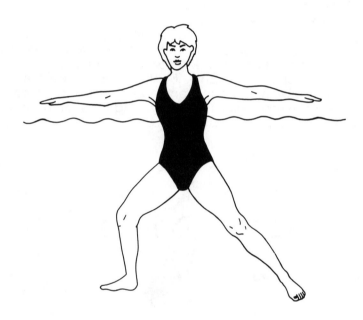

3. Pool-Wall Hamstring Stretch
Body part stretched: back of thigh (hamstrings).

Stand in chest-deep water, facing the pool wall. Grip the pool edge with both hands. Place the bottom of your right foot on the pool wall, keeping your leg straight. Your foot should be placed only at a point that you feel mild tension in the back of your thigh. Keep your back straight, so the stretch is all in your leg, not in your lower back. Hold the stretch. Relax. Repeat with your left leg.

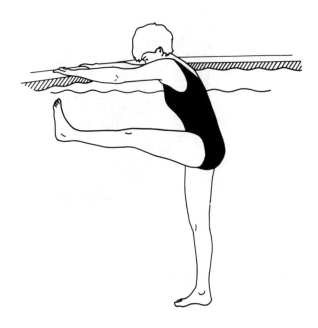

4. Hamstring Stretch on Pool Stairs
Body part stretched: back of thigh (hamstrings).

Stand facing the pool stairs. Rest your right heel on a step. Choose a height that is comfortable, not painful. You should feel mild tension in the back of your thigh. Keep your back straight and your arms relaxed and resting on the right leg. Hold the stretch. Relax. Repeat with your left leg.

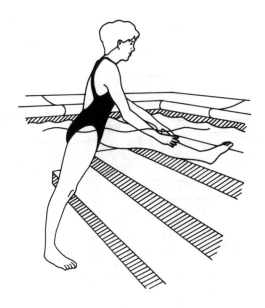

5. Front-of-Thigh Stretch
Body part stretched: front of thigh (quadriceps).

Stand in chest-deep water with your right side next to the pool wall. Hold the pool edge with right arm for balance. Bend your left knee, bringing your foot up behind you. Hold your left ankle with your left hand. Keep your back straight; don't try to increase the stretch by arching your lower back. Keep both knees side by side; don't let the left leg move forward or back in relation to your right leg. Hold the stretch. Relax. Repeat with your right leg, turning so your left side is next to the wall.

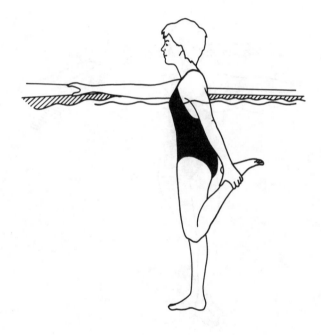

6. Hip Stretch

Body part stretched: outer hip (tensor fascia lata).

   Stand in chest-deep water with your left side facing the edge of the pool. Hold the pool wall with your left hand. Cross your left leg behind your right leg. Keeping both feet in place and flat on the pool bottom, lean your left hip toward the pool wall. Hold the stretch. Relax. Turn so your right side is facing the wall and repeat with the right hip.

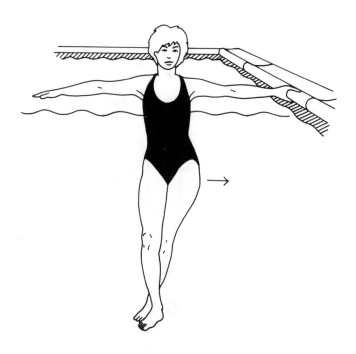

7. Side Stretch

Body part stretched: sides of torso (internal and external obliques); back (erector spinae).

   Stand in chest-deep water with your right side next to the pool wall. Rest your right arm on the pool edge for balance. Reach your left arm over your head, keeping the hips in place so the stretch is felt on the left side of your torso. Hold the stretch. Relax. Turn so your left side is facing the pool wall and repeat, this time stretching the right side.

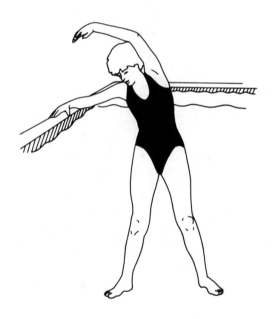

8. Cross-Body Shoulder Stretch

Body part stretched: shoulder (infraspinatus, posterior deltoid, teres major and minor); upper arm (triceps).

    Stand in the shallow end, grasp your right elbow with your
left hand, and gently pull your right arm across your chest.
Hold the stretch. Relax. Repeat, this time grasping your left
elbow with your right hand.

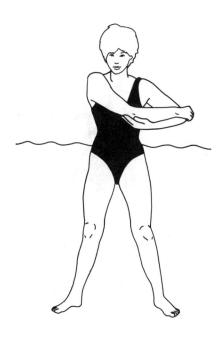

9. Behind-the-Head Shoulder Stretch

Body part stretched: shoulder (teres major, latissimus dorsi, posterior deltoid); upper arm (triceps).

Raise your right arm over your head. Bend it at the elbow so the hand drops behind your head. Grasp your right elbow with your left hand and gently pull your right arm toward the midline of your body. Hold the stretch. Relax. Repeat, this time grasping your left elbow with your right hand.

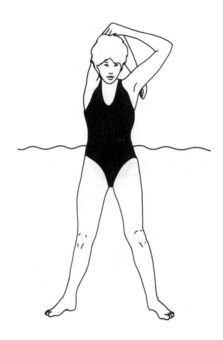

10. Neck Stretch

Body part stretched: neck (upper trapezius, neck flexors, and extensors).

Stand in the shallow end with your arms and shoulders relaxed. Gently bend your head to the left side, bringing it toward your left shoulder. Do not raise your shoulder to meet your head. Keep it relaxed. Close your eyes and breathe deeply as you hold the stretch. Return to the starting position. Repeat to the right.

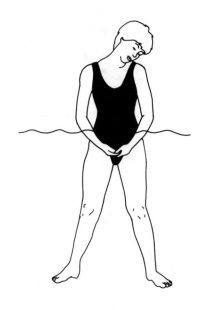

TOTAL-BODY STRETCHING WORKOUT

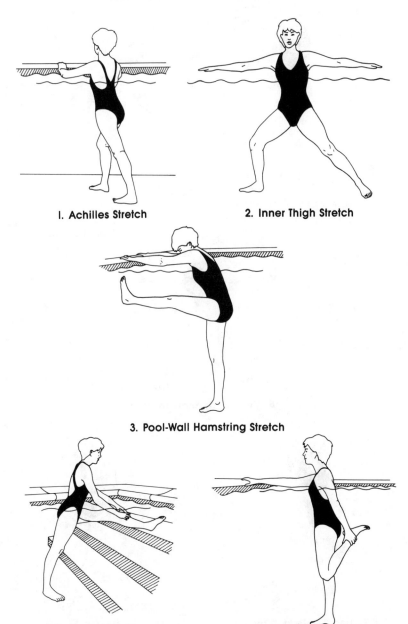

1. Achilles Stretch

2. Inner Thigh Stretch

3. Pool-Wall Hamstring Stretch

4. Hamstring Stretch on Pool Stairs

5. Front-of-Thigh Stretch

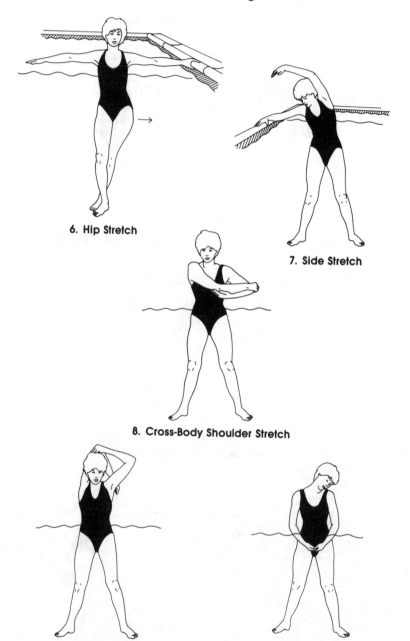

6. Hip Stretch

7. Side Stretch

8. Cross-Body Shoulder Stretch

9. Behind-the-Head Shoulder Stretch

10. Neck Stretch

WORKOUT SCHEDULE

Frequency: Stretch at the conclusion of your pool workout.
Duration: Hold each stretch for 10 to 30 seconds.
Intensity: Move to the position at which you feel mild tension in your muscles, never pain. Hold that position for the duration of the stretch, breathing slowly and deeply and concentrating on relaxation.

13
Water Workout Accessories

Throughout this book we have suggested many items to enhance your water workout recovery program. The following few pages offer you a guide to locating these accessories. We suggest where to buy them, what to look for in terms of quality, and approximately how much they will cost.

Most of these accessories are reasonably inexpensive and easy to find. We know that when you are injured, medical expenses can leave you with less money for "extras." Also, your injury may mean you're not feeling all that well, so you won't want to drive all over town looking for a special piece of water exercise equipment. We've selected items that should be easy to find and in some cases have listed a supplier's address and telephone number just in case the product is not available in your community.

These accessories will greatly enhance your workout and make it a lot easier to stick with it until you are back to normal. This especially applies to the flotation devices. If you have medical insurance and you are under the care of a physician or physical therapist your flotation device may be covered by the plan. Check with your insurance agent or the individual at your workplace who handles medical insurance claims.

Even if you must pay for the flotation device yourself, it is an important item to purchase, especially if you have a lower body or back injury. When you are well, you may want to continue doing deep-end running, in which case you will need the flotation device.

There are lots of gimmicks and "wonder products" on the market that claim to greatly improve your water workout. Our recovery program is designed so that in most cases your water workouts will be completed in a few weeks; and so we have stayed away from the gimmicks and kept the exercises as equipment free and convenient as possible. You can do almost every exercise in this book without using extra equipment. Even though this accessory list has been kept to a minimum, if you want to get the most from your program, we strongly suggest you look over this list. See if there is something that will make it that much easier for you to get in the pool and get well that much faster.

FLOTATION DEVICES

Waterskiing Belt or Waterskiing Vest

Belts are more comfortable to wear. They may be difficult to locate because they are not Coast Guard approved. Sporting goods stores may not have them in stock if they are not approved as flotation for waterskiing in your state. The vests may restrict your arm movement, but they are easier to locate. Try the vest on to be sure you can move your arms back and forth comfortably.

Where to shop: Check with sporting goods stores or

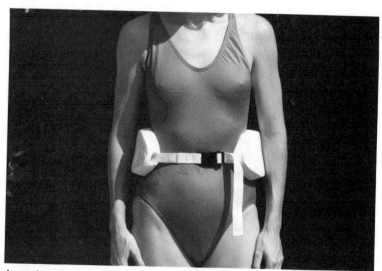

A waterskiing belt provides excellent flotation and allows your arms and shoulders freedom of movement.

stores specializing in waterskiing equipment. Retail outlets are listed in the telephone yellow pages under "sporting goods." Overton's Sports Center, a large mail-order sporting goods company, sells belts and vests. To obtain a catalog or to order, write or call: Overton's Sports Center, P.O. Box 8228, Greenville, North Carolina, USA 27835; (800) 334-6541; in North Carolina (800) 682-8263.

Price: Belts, $10 and up. Vests, $30 and up.

Wet Vest®

This product is manufactured especially for running workouts in the deep end of the pool. It allows you to stay submerged to neck level and gives you complete freedom of movement in the water. It comes in a variety of sizes, and for an additional charge you can have one custom-made. This is important if you are a large-sized, heavy individual since the waterskiing belt or waterski-

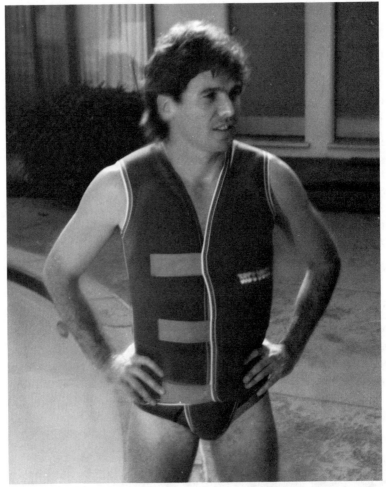

The Wet Vest® is specially designed for deep-end running.

ing vest may not provide you with sufficient flotation.

Where to shop: The Wet Vest can be ordered from the manufacturer. Write or call: Bioenergetics, Inc., 5074 Shelby Drive, Birmingham, Alabama, USA 35243; (800) 433-2627; in Alabama and Arkansas (205) 991-8842.

Price: $110 and up.

PORTABLE RADIO/CASSETTE PLAYER

Music will do a lot to pick up your spirits and keep you moving during the workout. Some of these products also have a clock with a second hand, which you can use to measure the seconds as you take your pulse or to time your workout. *Use only battery-operated radios or tape players near water. Plug-in appliances are not safe because of risk of electrical shock.*

Where to shop: Department stores and stores specializing in home electronics items are the best place to shop. Prices on these can vary a great deal from store to store, so watch the newspapers for sales or do some price checking on the phone.
Price: $20 and up.

WATER-RESISTANT WATCH

Watch manufacturers have been making sports watches that are water-resistant for many years. These days watches are usually digital and offer several sports-related features such as lap timing and a stop watch. You can use these watches to time the seconds

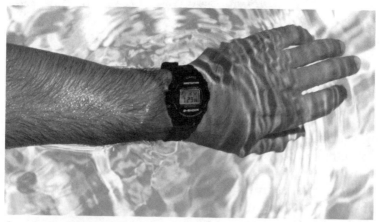

A water-resistant watch lets you take your pulse during an aerobic workout and time your exercise session.

while you take your pulse during an aerobic workout. They are also helpful in timing your exercise session, especially your warm-up and cool-down. Despite their many features, these watches are rather inexpensive.

Where to Shop: Department stores, sporting goods stores, scuba- and skin-diving specialty shops, and stores specializing in surfing equipment usually have these watches. Jewelry stores may carry some styles, but sports-oriented shops are your best bet.

Price: $25 and up.

HAND PADDLES

These are only for individuals with a wrist or elbow injury. They increase the resistance as you move your hand and forearm through the water. They are usually used by competitive swimmers during training.

Where to Shop: Some sporting goods stores carry these, especially if they have a special section with products for competitive swimming. The manager or coach of the local swim team may know a supplier in your commmunity.

Price: $6 to $10.

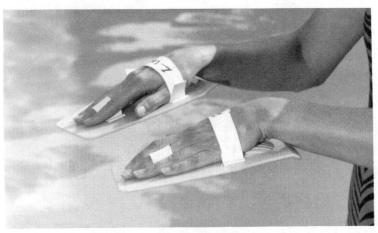

Hand paddles for wrist and elbow exercises.

KICK BOARDS

These simple, inexpensive pieces of foam will make your kicking exercises much easier. They are usually used by competitive swimmers during training sessions.

Where to shop: Sporting goods stores and shops specializing in equipment for competitive swimmers carry kick boards.

Price: $8 and up.

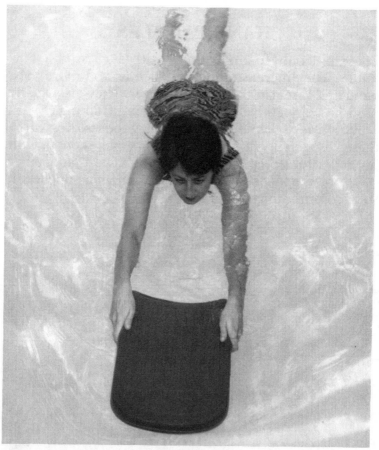

Kick boards provide important buoyancy for many lower body exercises.

BELT AND TETHER

This may be the toughest-to-find accessory on our list. This setup is only necessary if you are doing our deep-end sprinting workout. You can make your own, using a cloth belt with about twenty-five feet of surgical tubing looped through the back, or you can purchase one from the supplier we located.

Where to shop: Use a belt that fits snugly around your waist, as long as you don't mind getting it wet. Surgical tubing can be purchased at medical and hospital supply stores. Speed City, Inc., manufactures an excellent tether and belt system. It is called the Swimmer™ and is

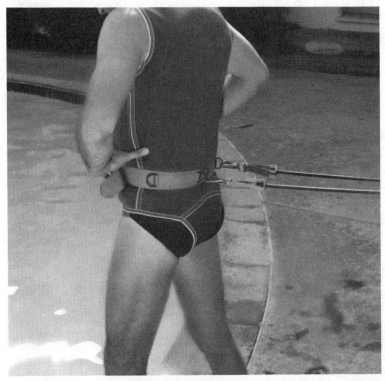

The Swimmer™, designed by Speed City, Inc., is a belt and tether that can be worn with a flotation device during your deep-end sprinting workout.

designed for use in the deep end. Write or telephone: Speed City, Inc., P.O. Box 1059, Portland, Oregon, USA 97207; (800) 255-9930, in Oregon (503) 684-5700.

Price: Surgical tubing for a homemade tether and belt, about 60¢ a foot. Speed City's Swimmer: about $50.

FINS

These are necessary only if you have a foot, ankle, or lower-leg injury. They are important because they make lower-leg kicking more challenging as you become stronger. Ask your friends if they have a pair of fins they can lend you. This is one of those items people

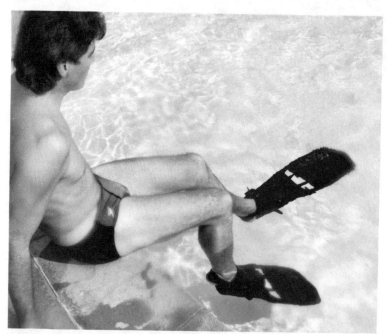

As your strength improves, swim fins make ankle exercises more challenging.

who like sports receive as gifts or buy and they aren't used all that often. There's a chance a friend has spare fins gathering dust in a closet. If you need to buy them, they are relatively inexpensive.

Where to shop: Sporting goods stores and shops specializing in scuba- and skin-diving equipment or surfing.

Price: $15 and up.

SNORKEL AND MASK

These accessories are only necessary if you have a back injury and are going to swim the freestyle. Wearing the mask and snorkel allows you to breathe without turning your head and spine.

Where to shop: Sporting goods stores and shops specializing in scuba- and skin-diving equipment.

Price: Snorkel, $5 and up. Mask, $15 and up.

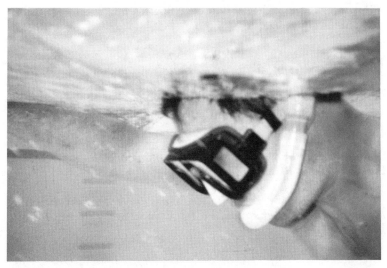

A snorkel and mask will allow you to breathe without turning your spine when you are swimming the freestyle.

References

Barham, J. N., and E. P. Wooten. *Structural Kinesiology.* New York: Macmillan, 1973.

Garrick, James G., and P. Radetsky. *Peak Condition: Winning Strategies to Prevent, Treat, and Rehabilitate Sports Injuries.* New York: Crown, 1986.

Kuland, D. N. *The Injured Athlete.* Philadelphia: J. B. Lippincott, 1982.

Morris, A. F. *Sports Medicine: Prevention of Athletic Injuries.* Dubuque: W. C. Brown, 1984.

Roy, S., and R. Irvin. *Sports Medicine: Prevention, Evaluation, Management, and Rehabilitation.* Englewood Cliffs: Prentice Hall, 1983.

Williams, J. M. *Applied Sport Psychology: Personal Growth to Peak Performance.* Palo Alto: Mayfield, 1986.

Index

Goals, setting of, in water
   recovery program, 26
Gracilis, 83
Guerrero, Lynnsey, 7

Hamstring strain or tear, 85
Hamstring stretch on pool
   stairs, 216, 223
Hand lifts, 164, 172
Hand paddles, 231
Heel spur, 42
Heyman, Steven R., 22
Hip extensions, 96, 101
Hip flexors, 83
Hip pain, outer, 87–88
Hip pointer, 88
Hip, thigh, and buttocks
   injuries
  anatomy, 82–84
  common, 85–90
  water exercise program
    for, 84–85, 90–101
   frog kicks, 97, 101
   hip extensions, 96, 101
   knee extensions, 94, 100
   leg circles, 92, 100
   leg curls, 93, 100
   scissors, 98, 102
   side leg lifts, 90, 99
   straight-leg kicks, 91, 99
   straight-leg raises, 95,
    101
   water cycling, 90, 99
  workout schedule for, 102
Hip stretch, 218, 224

Imagery, in water recovery
   program, 23
Impact injuries, 5
Infraspinatus, 132
Injury
  emotional side of, 20–21
  learning about, 33
  psychological pain of, 20
Inner thigh stretch, 214, 223

Interval training workouts,
   200–201
  workout schedule for,
   201–2, 209
Inward wrist turns, 168, 173

Johnstone, Jay, 6
Jumping jacks, 185, 203

Kennedy, John F., 1
Kick boards, 232–33
Kneecap, 61–62
Knee extensions, 70, 78, 94,
   100
knee lifts, 117, 128
Knee injuries
  anatomy, 60–62
  common, 63–66
  water exercise program
    for, 62–63, 67–80
   gentle knee kicks, 71, 78
   knee extensions, 70, 78
   lateral leg lifts, 74, 80
   leg curls, 69, 78
   scissors, 75, 80
   squats, 72, 79
   straight-leg kicks, 68, 77
   straight-leg walking, 67,
    77
   wall push-offs, 73, 79
   water cycling, 67, 77
  workout schedule for, 81
Knowledge, need for,
   concerning injury, 22–23
Kubler-Ross, Elizabeth, 20

Lateral ankle sprains, 43–44
Lateral epicondylitis, 155
Lateral leg lifts, 74, 80
Leg circles, 92, 100
Leg curls, 69, 78, 93, 100
Leg injuries. *See* Foot, ankle,
   and lower leg injuries;
   Hip, thigh, and buttock
   injuries